ONE HEALTH
and the Politics of
Antimicrobial Resistance

ONE HEALTH

and the Politics of

Antimicrobial Resistance

Laura H. Kahn, MD, MPH, MPP

Princeton University

JOHNS HOPKINS UNIVERSITY PRESS   BALTIMORE

© 2016 Johns Hopkins University Press
All rights reserved. Published 2016
Printed in the United States of America on acid-free paper
9 8 7 6 5 4 3 2 1

Johns Hopkins University Press
2715 North Charles Street
Baltimore, Maryland 21218-4363
www.press.jhu.edu

Library of Congress Cataloging-in-Publication Data

Kahn, Laura H., author.
  One Health and the politics of antimicrobial resistance /
Laura H. Kahn.
     p. ; cm.
  Includes bibliographical references and index.
  ISBN 978-1-4214-2004-2 (pbk. : alk. paper)—
ISBN 1-4214-2004-X (pbk. : alk. paper)—ISBN 978-1-4214-2005-9
(electronic)—ISBN 1-4214-2005-8 (electronic)
  I. Title.
  [DNLM: 1. One Health (Initiative) 2. Drug Resistance, Microbial.
3. International Cooperation. 4. Livestock. 5. Politics. 6. Poultry.
QW 45]
  QR46
  616.9'041—dc23   2015035547

A catalog record for this book is available from the British Library.

Special discounts are available for bulk purchases of this book. For more information, please contact Special Sales at 410-516-6936 or specialsales@press.jhu.edu.

Johns Hopkins University Press uses environmentally friendly book materials, including recycled text paper that is composed of at least 30 percent post-consumer waste, whenever possible.

Contents

CHAPTER ONE

The Politics

Antimicrobial resistance is a serious threat to human and animal health. Medical and public health leaders argue that the risks of nontherapeutic antibiotic use in livestock outweigh the benefits.[1] Veterinary medical and agricultural leaders insist that the benefits outweigh the risks. The cause for concern is that animal agriculture uses almost 80 percent of all antibiotics sold in the United States.[2] Intensive agriculture, for better or worse, has become as dependent on antibiotics as has modern medicine. This book examines the politics fueling this controversy.

For years, the US agriculture lobby has successfully fought legislation that would restrict nontherapeutic antibiotic use in livestock and poultry production.[3] The American Farm Bureau Federation (AFBF), the self-described "Voice of Agriculture," opposes the proposed legislation, the Preservation of Antibiotics for Medical Treatment Act, because it believes that no public health threat has arisen after 40 years of nontherapeutic antibiotic use in livestock. The AFBF asserts that limiting nontherapeutic antibiotic use in livestock would have negative economic and animal-health consequences.[4]

The Alliance for the Prudent Use of Antibiotics (APUA) blames part of the spread of antibiotic-resistant microbes on the widespread use of nontherapeutic antibiotics in livestock and wants the practice banned. In *The Antibiotic Paradox*, Dr. Stuart B. Levy, professor of medicine at Tufts University School of Medicine and president and founder of APUA, wrote, "Given legislative politics, better-educated consumers will demand animals free of human antibiotic consumption. Only then will we see definitive changes."[5]

The conflict between medicine and agriculture is well illustrated by a *New York Times* article covering a report about retail meat published by the National Antimicrobial Resistance Monitoring System (NARMS), a surveillance system run collaboratively by the Centers for Disease Control and Prevention (CDC), the Food and Drug Administration (FDA), and the Department of

Agriculture (USDA).[6,] On April 16, 2013, Stephanie Strom's article appeared and described the political clash that ensued after the FDA released the 2011 NARMS report. Published in early 2013, the report received little attention until the Environmental Working Group (EWG), an environmental research and advocacy organization partly supported by Applegate, a company that sells organic and antibiotic-free meat, released its report, "Superbugs Invade American Supermarkets," which was based on the NARMS findings.[7] The EWG report stated that industrial livestock producers misuse antibiotics, spawning multi-drug-resistant superbugs, which together cause 3.6 million cases of food poisoning per year. Veterinarians working with the International Food Information Council, a nonprofit organization financed partly by large food corporations and the US Farmers and Ranchers Alliance, criticized EWG's report as deceptive.

Strom's article about the politics of antimicrobial resistance generated its own heated exchange. In a letter to the editor, Dr. Bernadette Dunham, director of the Center for Veterinary Medicine at the FDA, wrote, "Describing bacteria that are resistant to one, or even a few, drugs as 'superbugs' is inappropriate. . . . It is critical that we continue to minimize antimicrobial resistance and promote appropriate and judicious use of antimicrobials in both humans and animals."[8] Congresswoman Louise M. Slaughter, a microbiologist, representative of New York's 25th district, and a sponsor of the Preservation of Antibiotics for Medical Treatment Act, responded, "I am astonished by the letter from Bernadette Dunham. . . . The FDA itself said in 1977 that feeding antibiotics . . . to farm animals indiscriminately was dangerous to human health. . . . The FDA, tasked with protecting the public's health, should understand that, given the 70,000 deaths a year that are due to antibiotic-resistant infections."[9]

As the controversy continues, the CDC estimates that more than 1 million people in the United States are sickened annually from bacterial foodborne diseases. Of the top five pathogens causing people to be hospitalized with foodborne illness, approximately 50 percent are due to three bacterial species commonly present in livestock and poultry: nontyphoidal *Salmonella, Campylobacter* species, and *Escherichia coli* (STEC) 0157.[10] Many of these bacteria are resistant to at least one antibiotic.[11] The agriculture lobby insists that proper food preparation, handling, and cooking make the risk of disease transmission negligible.

The ongoing debate regarding the level of risk to human health of the nontherapeutic use of antibiotics in livestock defines the politics of antimicrobial resistance and provides the rationale for this book. Antibiotic use in plant agriculture, constituting about 0.12 percent of total antibiotic use in agriculture, has been less controversial and is not discussed here. Companion animals can serve as potential reservoirs of antibiotic-resistant microbes; however, their use has not been politicized and is minimally covered.[12] My goal in this book is to investigate the use of antibiotics and antimicrobial resistance in food animals and humans, integrating the perspectives of medicine, public health, veterinary medicine, and agriculture. The One Health concept serves as an analytic framework.

The One Health concept recognizes that human, animal, and environmental health are inextricably linked; because they are linked, interdisciplinary solutions are needed.[13] A One Health approach is important because the popular press has been severely critical of livestock producers, driving them to become defensive and adversarial and reducing opportunities for open and honest dialogue and cooperation. Understanding the politics requires examining the history, economics, sociology, and science surrounding antibiotic use and resistance in humans and animals.

One Health

One Health is a new term with ancient roots. Hippocrates, the Greek physician (460–370 BCE), recognized the impact of environmental conditions on human health in his *On Airs, Waters, and Places*.[14] He knew that certain environments, such as swampy, stagnant waters, made people sick. Around two thousand years passed before scientists discovered that mosquitoes transmit malaria, which literally means "bad air."

Unfortunately, the recognition of the interconnectedness of human, animal, and environmental health was largely lost during the Middle Ages and not rediscovered until after the Renaissance. For example, in eighteenth-century England, contemporary folklore posited that milkmaids who got cowpox never developed smallpox. Dr. Edward Jenner, a young physician, decided to test this folklore and developed a smallpox vaccine from the dried pus of cowpox vesicles.[15] Jenner derived the term "vaccine" from the Latin word "vacca," meaning cow.[16] Two centuries later, public health officials used a purified form of this same vaccine to eradicate naturally occurring smallpox.

Drs. Louis Pasteur and Robert Koch developed the germ theory of disease by studying, respectively, silkworm diseases and anthrax, a bacterial disease of livestock.[17] Pasteur discovered the field of immunology by studying chicken cholera. He found that chicken cholera broth that had been sitting unused in a flask for a month did not kill chickens after they were injected with it. Subsequent injections with fresh broth did not kill them either. The "old" broth had made them immune. Pasteur correctly surmised that the bacteria had become attenuated over time and boosted the chickens' ability to fight the disease. This insight provided the basis for the development of future vaccines.[18]

Drs. Theobald Smith and F. L. Kilbourne, a physician-veterinarian team, discovered that arthropods (e.g., insects) could transmit disease. They were studying cattle fever when they found that ticks spread *Babesia bigemina,* the parasite responsible for the disease. *B. bigemina* primarily infects domestic and wild animals but occasionally infects humans. The parasite invades red blood cells and can cause a malaria-type illness. Their monumental work set the stage for Walter Reed and his colleagues to discover that mosquitoes spread yellow fever.[19] One could argue that many of the greatest discoveries in the history of medicine and public health were made at the junction between human and animal health.

Unfortunately, the synergistic collaborative efforts between the professions waned as the twentieth century progressed. Medicine became increasingly specialized and reductionistic in its approach to health and disease, forgetting about the important contributions of veterinary medicine. Support for comparative medicine, the study of disease processes across species, also waned, reducing research opportunities for veterinarians.[20]

The history of antibiotics' discovery and impact on human health has been well documented. Less well known is how and why antibiotics became an integral part of agriculture, particularly in food-animal production. This book briefly examines the history and economics of food-animal production in the United States as well as the history behind the European ban on the use of nontherapeutic antibiotics.

The European Experience

Unlike the United States and other nations, European countries have been aggressive in restricting nontherapeutic antibiotic use in livestock. In the late 1960s, the British government examined the controversial use of nontherapeutic antibiotics in livestock after experiencing a series of antibiotic-resistant *Salmonella typhimurium* outbreaks. The Swann Report, published in 1969, recommended that antibiotics important for human use not be used for growth promotion purposes in livestock, but that they should be used to prevent disease and treat sick animals.[21] Political opposition hindered Parliament's implementation of most of the report's recommendations.

Almost 20 years later, Sweden became the first country to ban the nontherapeutic use of antibiotics in livestock. The Swedish farmers not only supported the ban; they instigated it. In the late 1990s, Denmark introduced a similar ban in response to the emergence of vancomycin-resistant enterococcus (VRE). Concerns about VRE and other resistant infections drove the European Union, in 2006, to ban all nontherapeutic antibiotic use in livestock in all member nations. The European Union passed the ban despite opposition from the Scientific Community on Animal Nutrition, a panel of animal health experts.[22] Understanding the experiences in these countries, and in Europe as a whole, after the bans went into effect is vital for informed policymaking and is a central focus of this book.

The US Experience

For decades, the US Food and Drug Administration has been grappling with the dilemma of nontherapeutic antibiotic use in livestock. In 1970, in response to the United Kingdom's Swann Report, the FDA Scientific Advisory Committee recommended establishing a task force to review the issue. Two years later, the task force released its report, finding that low levels of antibiotics in animal feed favored the development of antibiotic-resistant bacteria and that human illnesses and deaths had resulted from antibiotic-resistant bacteria of animal origin, such as *Salmonella*. The task force recommended restricting the use in livestock of antibiotics having important use in human medicine.[23]

Responding to the recommendations, the FDA planned to hold hearings with the intent of restricting the use of penicillins and tetracyclines as growth promoters. But the farm industry lobbied Congress to stop the FDA, and as a result, the agency ceased all efforts to restrict the use of growth-promoting antibiotics. Thirty years later, consumer advocacy groups petitioned the agency to reconsider the issue. The FDA issued voluntary guidelines to livestock producers and pharmaceutical companies.[24] US policymakers largely passed the tough decisions regarding nontherapeutic antibiotic use in livestock to consumers, who had to decide whether they were willing to pay more for "organically grown" antibiotic-free animal products. In fall 2014 the White House issued a national strategy to combat antimicrobial resistance, supporting the FDA's voluntary measures for limiting the use of medically important antibiotics in livestock and advocating for a One Health approach in disease surveillance.[25]

International Challenges

Antimicrobial resistance is an international problem. Highlighting the seriousness of the issue, on April 7, 2011, the World Health Organization (WHO) dedicated World Health Day to antimicrobial resistance and stressed the urgent need for action. According to Bernard Vallat, director-general of the World Organisation for Animal Health, more than 100 countries are without legislation controlling antibiotic use in humans or livestock.[26]

The situation has become dire. Some intestinal bacteria that commonly cause infections, such as *E. coli,* have acquired mobile genes conferring resistance to virtually all antibiotics, including carbapenem, the antibiotic of last resort. WHO has urged policymakers to strengthen disease surveillance, improve laboratory capacity, regulate and control the appropriate use of antibiotics, and foster innovation and research for new diagnostics and treatment options.[27]

In 2014 WHO released a report showing the extent and severity of antimicrobial resistance and warned that the world was approaching a "post-antibiotic era." A *New York Times* editorial stated that unregulated antibiotic use, together with poor sanitation and health care, have fueled the rise of resistant bacteria.[28] It singled out India for creating "the perfect breeding ground" for bacteria resistant to virtually all antibiotics. The editorial also blamed the overuse of antibiotics in livestock as the cause for antibiotic resistance in the United States.

As the effectiveness of many antibiotics diminishes, global demand for meat and other animal products increases. The UN Food and Agriculture Organization's (FAO's) 2011 World Livestock Report estimates that from 2010 to 2050 total global meat consumption will increase by almost 73 percent; global consumption of poultry is expected to increase by 125 percent. In developing countries, increases in consumption during the next 40 years are estimated to be even steeper than in developed countries. Total meat consumption in developing countries is anticipated to increase more than 100 percent, and for poultry alone, to increase by almost 180 percent.[29] According to the FAO, the world will need an additional 1,305 million tons of grain by 2050, of which 60 percent will feed humans directly and 40 percent will feed livestock. Much of the extra demand for livestock feed will be in poultry and pork production.[30] The effects of the bans on the nontherapeutic use of antibiotics in livestock production in Europe will be an important part of the One Health analysis.

Environmental Challenges

New scientific discoveries suggest that antibiotic-resistant genes are not a new phenomenon in response to extensive human use, but rather are ancient and ubiquitous. These resistance genes form a global "resistome." Extensive antibiotic use in humans and animals has placed intense selective pressures on microbes to express their resistance genes in order to survive. Many resistance genes persist in manure and wastewater sludge; when those substances are applied to agricultural fields, the resistance genes become integrated with soil microbes. Wildlife, especially birds, help transmit resistance genes around the world.

Antibiotics are used in both terrestrial and aquatic agriculture. Fish farms help mitigate the depletion of the world's oceans but present unique challenges. Antibiotics are not used for growth promotion but rather for disease prevention in fish raised in densely populated environments. Antibiotic residues on fish sold in markets have been detected.

Antibiotics affect microbes not only in global environments but also in internal environments: the microbiomes. The Human Microbiome Project has revealed that the human body is primarily made up of bacterial cells.[31] Understanding the impact of antibiotics on microbiomes is an area of active research, shedding new light on our understanding of health and disease.

Pharmaceutical Hurdles

Complicating the antibiotic resistance problem further, the pipeline for new antibiotics has largely dried up. The "golden age" of antibiotic development lasted from the 1940s to the 1960s; during that period new classes of chemicals with antibacterial properties were developed and produced. Unfortunately, microbial expression of antibiotic-resistant genes appeared almost as soon as new drugs became available for clinical use.[32]

In the 1990s, the pharmaceutical industry developed countermeasures against resistant microbes primarily by modifying preexisting antibiotics. Since then, it has largely lost interest in developing new antibiotics. Costs for research and development have been greater than the returns. Compared to drugs that treat chronic diseases, antibiotics yield low returns, because they are used for short periods of time. The FDA has not helped the situation by creating regulatory hurdles for approving new antibiotics.[33] Professional medical organizations, such as the Infectious Diseases Society of America (IDSA), have been urging Congress to pass legislation providing incentives for drug companies to develop new antibiotics.

Political Engagement and Commitment

The use of nontherapeutic antibiotics in livestock presents a far more complex issue than has been portrayed in the media. There is no question that antimicrobial resistance poses a tremendous threat to human and animal health. No one argues that the indiscriminate use of antibiotics is not harmful, but addressing the problem has been difficult because the subject has become so politicized. At stake are not only the future of modern medicine but also the future of modern agriculture.

As global antibiotic resistance worsens, the challenge of sustainably meeting the growing world population's demands for meat and dairy products intensifies. Meeting the growing demand for animal protein will be difficult without intensive livestock production. As it is, global food production has yet to feed everyone: in 2010 almost 1 billion people suffered from chronic hunger and undernutrition.[34] The United Nations estimates that by 2050 the world's population will increase to approximately 9 billion, assuming fertility rates continue at mid-estimated levels.[35] Producing affordable meat for the world's poor in the presence of climate change, water shortages, emerging diseases, and increasing feed costs will make livestock production ever more challenging, requiring an increase in the efficiency of converting animal feed into healthy animals for human consumption.

Intensive livestock production promotes food security (i.e., access to nutritious food) by allowing the poor to afford meat and dairy products. Beef raised in intensive agricultural systems costs about one-third of the price of beef raised on grassland pastures. Food-insecure families cannot afford to buy grass-fed beef. Although animal protein is not necessary for human survival, it is highly beneficial because of the nutrients it provides.[36]

Affluent, developed nations have strong and growing consumer movements opposed to intensive agriculture. Books such as *Diet for a Small Planet, The Omnivore's Dilemma, Food Matters,* and *Eating Animals* discuss the hazards of modern agriculture and advocate changing eating behaviors, including eating less meat. These efforts have helped raise awareness of the finite nature of the planet's natural resources for food production. Corporate food chains are responding to the public's concerns. In 2003 the McDonald's Corporation, the world's largest restaurant chain, asked its meat suppliers to reduce their use of antibiotics in livestock.[37]

We must get the balance right between the need for safe, effective antibiotics and the need for safe, affordable meat and dairy products to ensure the public's health and well-being. Farmers and veterinarians must be considered part of the solution, not part of the problem; they must support government policies, not oppose them, in order for those policies to be effective.

The One Health analysis in this book is evidenced based. More than 90 related charts and figures are available at www.press.jhu.edu for readers to examine, and to inform class discussions. An asterisk at the end of a sentence indicates one or more corresponding charts or figures on the designated Johns Hopkins University Press website.

Ultimately, the goal for both public health and agriculture should be to optimize human, animal, and environmental health: in essence, One Health. Advances in science and technology will help address these challenges, but such advances take time to develop and implement. Until then, preserving the effectiveness of antibiotics while continuing to provide animal proteins to the world's growing population will require political engagement and commitment.

CHAPTER TWO

A Brief History of Meat Production and Antibiotics

The heart of the controversy between medicine and agriculture revolves around humanity's demand for meat and other animal products. Philosophers have been concerned for centuries with the problems associated with eating meat. The ancient Greek philosopher Socrates (470–399 BCE) believed that wars were caused by the quest for new territories to meet food animals' extensive need for grazing land. Eighteenth-century British philosophers William Paley (1743–1805) and Robert Malthus (1766–1834) wrote about the extravagance and environmental wastefulness of raising food animals. In the twentieth and twenty-first centuries, philosophers have added animal welfare and suffering to the concerns about meat production and consumption.[1] However, without the domestication of plants and animals, civilization would not exist.

There are inherent disease risks associated with eating meat. For example, genetic evidence suggests that the measles virus diverged from the rinderpest virus, a disease of cattle, sometime between the eleventh and twelfth centuries. Eating meat from wild animals presents different disease risks.[2] Yet, despite these problems, meat is a fundamental part of many people's diets. Indeed, some have argued that we evolved into modern humans *because* we hunted, cooked, and ate animals.[3] Eating meat is deeply embedded in many cultures, especially in the United States.

Not only did the early colonists of North America find a continent rich with wildlife; they also brought their cattle, sheep, and pigs with them from Europe. These early Americans enjoyed a meat-centric diet that their poor brethren back in England could only dream about. In much of Europe, only the wealthy and ruling classes could afford to eat meat on a regular basis.[4]

Manifest destiny pushed livestock production across North America. During the nineteenth century, cowboys on horseback drove millions of head of cattle across the western plains to stockyards in Kansas, Illinois, and Missouri en route to feed the city-dwellers along the East Coast. Meat production, particularly the slaughter of animals, moved outside of cities and became invisible to urbanites.[5] As a result, cities became much cleaner, benefiting public health.

In the early 1900s, bad weather and exceptionally poor corn crops contributed to high meat prices. The public blamed the meat companies. President Theodore Roosevelt assigned James Garfield, son of former president James A. Garfield, to investigate. Garfield verified that the high meat prices were the result of crop failures and high corn prices, not corporate schemes or conspiracies.[6] But this finding did not diminish consumers' complaints about the high cost of living.[7]

In 1905 a series of reports in *Lancet* exposed poorly ventilated, unsanitary, and inhumane conditions in the Chicago stockyards and meatpacking houses.[8] Upton Sinclair's incendiary novel *The Jungle* about the same subject fueled public outrage. One year later, *Lancet* editors congratulated themselves and the public for bringing the scandal to the attention of the president of the United States.[9] Congress was forced to act and passed the 1906 Food and Drug Act. (Additional information about this and subsequent legislation, as it relates to antibiotics, appears in chapter 7.)

Before the United States entered World War I, meat prices were high, because outdated production methods could not meet the demands of growing urban populations. Poor weather, crop diseases, and increased food purchases by the British, French, and Italian governments added to the problem. The Europeans faced severe food shortages. Their herds were slaughtered, and meat production dwindled as the war raged on.[10]

Germany particularly suffered during World War I because it had become dependent on imported animal fodder to feed its expanding livestock population. The German government took virtually no action, for example, establishing national grain stores, to prepare for the inevitable shortages resulting from economic blockades imposed by the Allies.[11] With a shortage of food, regional and local German officials focused on providing survival rations of bread and potatoes to the public. But rather than grow more grain, German farmers preferred to raise meat and produce dairy products, because these were highly coveted and sold for more money on the black market.[12] By the end of the war, food accounted for half of German workers' household expenditures, and women and children were protesting in the streets.[13]

In the United States, poor Americans living in the tenements of Boston, New York, and Philadelphia protested the high prices of food by looting grocery stores and fighting with police. Housewives and bakers joined forces and demanded a cessation of food exports to Europe. When the United States declared war, the National Agricultural Organization, a newly formed activist organization, contacted thousands of newspaper editors to support a federal guarantee on the price of food. President Woodrow Wilson wavered. The nation's farmers were opposed to price fixing, but the public demanded action.[14]

President Wilson reluctantly agreed to a temporary wartime food administration that would stimulate production, protect consumers from high prices, regulate distribution, conserve food, and eliminate waste. Congress approved the controversial emergency measure, the Lever Food Control Act of August 1917.[15] Herbert Hoover, a "food expert" based on his leadership of the Commission for Relief in Belgium, an organization that directed food to German-occupied Belgium, agreed to lead the agency.[16]

The president called on the nation's farmers to increase production, since "a nation in arms" also meant farmers in arms. The farmers responded by taking out loans to buy more land, animals, and supplies to build barns and silos. Meat production increased; from 1917 to 1919, pork production rose approximately 20 percent.[17]

When the war ended, US food surpluses were sent to Europe to avert starvation there. American farmers, flush with cash from wartime income, paid exorbitant prices for farm equipment and expensive purebred livestock. By the fall of 1919, Europeans could no longer afford to buy American meat. Pork prices and, to a lesser extent, beef prices dropped precipitously. Farmers could not believe that their efforts to ease starvation abroad and curb high prices at home would lead to plummeting prices. The Federal Reserve System, which had been set up to address such crises, ignored their calls for help.[18]

Congress moved slowly to confront the problem. In 1924 and 1927, President Calvin Coolidge vetoed the McNary-Haugen bill, which would have established tariff protections and set up a federal export corporation to sell surplus food on the international market. He was opposed to price fixing and to creating a new federal "cancerous bureaucracy."[19]

President Herbert Hoover was more supportive of the farmers' plight. In 1929 he signed the Agricultural Marketing Act, which authorized $500 million for agricultural cooperatives to purchase price-suppressing surpluses and keep them off the market.[20] Unfortunately, this effort was too little and too late.

The US farm crisis from 1919 to 1923 was followed by a severe drought in the Midwest, bringing more disaster to farmers. Many farmers went bankrupt and abandoned their farms. In the decade between 1910 and 1920, the percentage of people living in urban areas surpassed that of people living in rural areas for the first time in US history.*[21]

In 1935 wind erosion of parched farmland caused devastating dust storms, ruined crops, and killed livestock. The southern Great Plains, including Kansas, New Mexico, Colorado, and the panhandles of Texas and Oklahoma, were primarily affected; the region became known as the "Dust Bowl." The Great Depression was the final blow. Food prices collapsed. From 1929 to 1932, pork prices fell 165 percent. Beef prices fell 100 percent.*[22]

In 1933 the newly elected President Franklin D. Roosevelt, together with Democratic majorities in Congress, passed legislation providing economic relief to farmers. The Agricultural Adjustment Act created the Agricultural Adjustment Administration (AAA), which, in an attempt to restore parity purchasing power, paid farmers to limit the production of seven commodities: cotton, corn, dairy products, hogs, rice, tobacco, and wheat. The legislation had unintended consequences. A pork surplus that year led to the unfortunate AAA decision to pay farmers to slaughter 6 million piglets rather than glut the market. Henry A. Wallace, the secretary of agriculture, responded to criticisms about the slaughter in the face of widespread hunger by stating that farmers could not "run an old folks home for hogs and keep them around indefinitely as barnyard pets."[23]

Additional New Deal legislation and the onset of World War II fundamentally changed the federal government's relationship with agriculture through regulation and economic aid. Five million people left farms for better-paying jobs in cities or for military service; they were replaced by combines, corn pickers, and tractors. These changes benefited large-scale enterprises; small family farms could not compete. Farming became strictly a business, an increasingly technical and efficient place to work and less a way of life.[24]

The United States implemented food rationing from 1942 to 1946.[25] Meat, especially beef, was sent to the soldiers. The civilian population had to eat lower-quality cuts of meat, fish, pork, and poultry—but their fare was still better than what the Europeans had. The British survived on less than half the American rations. A black market focused on meat emerged. Small slaughterhouses evaded inspectors from the Office of Price Administration. The illegal trade in meat threatened the ability of the United States to provide enough meat to Great Britain.[26]

After the war, meat prices continued to climb. From 1942 to 1948, beef prices increased almost 125 percent. The price for broiler chickens increased 57 percent.* Desperate to increase production and bring down meat prices, the US government increased funding for animal feed and nutrition research.[27]

Animal proteins, such as cod liver oil and fishmeal, help livestock, including chickens and pigs, build muscle tissue. Without these products, the animals are prone to disease and weigh less at maturity—meaning less meat for consumption. Plant-derived proteins are not effective substitutes. Before World War II, Norway provided cod liver oil and Japan provided fishmeal to American farmers. The war stopped these suppliers: Germany invaded Norway and the United States declared war on Japan. Academic, corporate, and USDA researchers struggled to find substitutes for these products.[28]

In 1948 Thomas H. Jukes, a biochemist at Lederle Laboratories in New York, a division of American Cyanamid Company, was researching vitamin B12 as a supplement for poultry raised on vegetable proteins, such as soybean meal. He accidentally discovered that feed fermented with *Streptomyces aureofaciens* (a microorganism used to make chlortetracycline [aureomycin]) resulted in a dramatic increase in weight and decrease in mortality. Chicks fed 300 ml per kilogram of aureomycin in their feed for 25 days grew on average two-and-a-half-times heavier than control chicks and had a mortality rate of 8 percent compared to an average mortality rate of 83 percent in the two control groups. The group fed high doses of liver extract grew almost as well as the high-dose aureomycin group and had the same 8 percent mortality rate. Follow-up studies confirmed the findings (fig. 2.1).[29]

The results were so impressive that two years later, the commercial feeding of low-dose antibiotics to chicks, piglets, and calves began. The first antibiotics included chlortetracycline, oxytetracycline, penicillin, and streptomycin. Bacitracin and tylosin soon followed. The doses were originally 50 grams per ton of feed (about 50 ppm), but levels as high as 200 ppm were often used. Jukes was aware of the development of resistant organisms. He wrote,

> From the first, it was evident that the feeding of antibiotics produced resistant microorganisms in the digestive tract because the surviving organisms have to tolerate antibiotics. Some typical experiments showed a temporary drop in

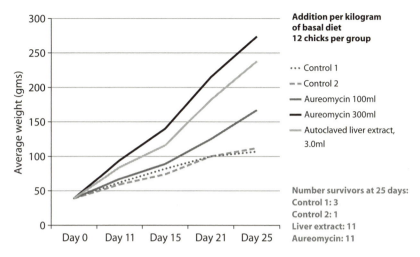

Fig. 2.1. Effect of aureomycin (chlortetracycline) on chick growth. *Source:* T. H. Jukes, "Public Health Significance of Feeding Low Levels of Antibiotics to Animals," *Advances in Applied Microbiology* 16 (1973): 1–30, data abstracted from table 1, p. 2.

numbers of intestinal bacteria for the first day or two, followed by a return to levels higher than before. What we were not prepared for was the fact that the changed and resistant flora were in some way beneficial, due either to the presence of certain new bacterial strains or the absence of certain former strains or species . . . the growth effect is so illogical that I recommend others trying the experiment with chicks.[30]

The benefits were seen not only in chicks, but in ill and malnourished children as well. In 1957 African children with marasmus, a form of severe malnutrition, showed marked improvement compared to controls after two to seven weeks of low-dose chlortetracycline.[31] A more recent study (2009–11) of severely malnourished children in Malawi found similarly beneficial results. The study was criticized for potentially inducing antimicrobial resistance; alternative strategies such as safe drinking water and improved hygiene were recommended.[32]

The use of low-dose antibiotics in livestock, especially pigs and poultry, was widely adopted. Production increased and prices decreased in the United States. From 1950 to 1960, the price per pound of broiler chickens decreased 38 percent: during the 1960s, the average price per pound was 14.8 cents. The price remained low until inflation hit in 1973.[33]

Americans enjoyed relatively inexpensive food. After 1950, the share of disposable income that Americans spent on food decreased approximately 50 percent. In 2000 the percentage dropped below 10 percent for the first time.* Food shortages and high prices became a concern of poor, developing countries such as Cambodia and Chad, where the percent of income spent on food can be over 80 percent.[34]

Unfortunately, at the same time farmers began feeding antibiotics to livestock, antibiotic-resistant microbes began appearing in postwar Japanese patients. Outbreaks of sulfonamide-resistant shigella dysentery led Japanese scientists to discover that multiple drug resistances could be transferred between bacteria as "infective heredity." Various derivatives of sulfonamides had been introduced in Japan at the end of the war to treat bacillary dysentery, a type of severe diarrhea. The sulfonamides were highly effective for several years, until resistance developed. To counter the growing problem, newer antibiotics such as streptomycin, tetracycline, and chloramphenicol were substituted; however, within four years, after 1957, resistance to these antibiotics appeared as well. In 1959, after researching the problem, Japanese scientists concluded that multiple-drug-resistant genes could be transferred from resistant bacteria (e.g., shigellae) to sensitive bacteria (e.g., *Escherichia coli*) by conjugation (bacterial mating and sharing of genetic material) while mixing within the intestines of patients. Conjugation could occur both within bacterial species and between species. Tsutomu Watanabe, a bacteriologist at the Keio University School of Medicine in Tokyo, reviewed the Japanese experience and concluded, presciently, that antimicrobial resistance could become a serious global problem.[35]

CHAPTER THREE

The British Experience

During the mid-1960s, Dr. Ephraim Saul Anderson, the director of the British Enteric Reference Laboratory (ERL), noticed an increase in *Salmonella typhimurium* infections in calves. These infections appeared soon after farmers adopted intensive farming methods. Dr. Anderson believed the intensive rearing of calves caused these infections.[1]

The new animal-husbandry practices involved separating calves from their mothers shortly after birth. They were subsequently transported over long distances, with many other newborn calves from different breeders, to crowded facilities where they were retained for several months before being passed to dealers or markets, or both. Mixing and congregating calves from different breeders provided perfect opportunities for pathogens, especially *S. typhimurium* type 29, to cross and spread.[2]

Many of the animals became infected with *S. typhimurium,* developed infectious diarrhea, and died. Bacterial specimens sent to the ERL grew an increasing proportion of *S. typhimurium* type 29 resistant to streptomycin and sulfonamide.[3] The organism subsequently developed resistance to other antibiotics as well, including ampicillin, furazolidone, kanamycin, neomycin, and tetracyclines.

Dr. Anderson attributed some of the spread of organisms resistant to furazolidone, a nitrofuran antibiotic with a broad spectrum activity against Gram-positive and -negative organisms, to one particular dealer who distributed the antibiotic to his clients with instructions to administer it to the calves for several weeks to prevent infectious diarrhea. He did not know when the dealer began this practice, but he noted that *S. typhimurium* type 29 resistant to furazolidone appeared in November 1964 and rapidly increased in prevalence thereafter. This dealer distributed calves receiving furazolidone to many parts of the United Kingdom, spreading resistant *S. typhimurium* type

29 with them. Around the country, outbreaks in calves caused by *S. typhimurium* type 29 could be traced back to the same dealer.[4]

The majority of animal cultures growing resistant *S. typhimurium* type 29 came from calves raised in crowded conditions. Sick animals had to be treated with antibiotics to fight infections; healthy animals were given antibiotics to prevent infections. Furazolidone was the most commonly used drug to prevent and treat infectious diarrhea in cattle.[5]

In 1965 the ERL received 1,297 bovine (mostly calves) and 576 human cultures of infections with *S. typhimurium* type 29. Of these, 99.7 percent of the bovine and 96.5 percent of the human cultures were antibiotic-resistant. Six people died from these infections. The human infections were usually associated with animals in some way, such as in farm workers and their families or veterinary workers handling calves.[6]

An outbreak of gastroenteritis involving *S. typhimurium* type 29 sickened 59 people who consumed raw milk from dairy cows infected with the organism. The farmer in charge of the dairy had recently begun the practice of intensive calf rearing and had imported very young calves from a dealer more than 100 miles away. Some of the calves died from diarrhea. The Veterinary Investigation Service of the Ministry of Agriculture, Fisheries, and Food (MAFF) subsequently determined the cause to be *S. typhimurium*. Dr. V. P. Geoghegan, the medical officer of Midhurst Rural District reporting the human outbreak, noted that salmonellosis in cattle was not a reportable disease, so that if an outbreak were occurring in dairy cattle, the responsible medical officer would not necessarily know about it. The primary reason he knew about the outbreak at the dairy farm was that he had an excellent relationship with the Divisional Veterinary Surgeon who had informed him.[7]

But aside from the resistant *S. typhimurium* type 29 outbreaks in cattle and humans, it was not clear whether other microbes were becoming resistant from the feeding of antibiotics to livestock. Dr. Anderson wrote, "With the exception of the clearly defined instances of human infection with drug-resistant *S. typhimurium,* I do not know to what extent drug resistance is of animal origin, and unless we can find a method of distinguishing R [resistance] factors arising in the bacteria of animals from those arising in the bacteria of man we shall have no exact information on this subject."[8]

Outbreaks of resistant *S. typhimurium* from cattle to humans and increasing concern over drug-resistant *Escherichia coli* infections in humans prompted the Netherthorpe Committee, a joint advisory committee to the Agricultural and Medical Research Councils, to recommend in July 1968 that a new advisory committee be assembled to address these developing concerns.[9] In response, the Health and Agriculture ministers appointed the Joint Committee on the Use of Antibiotics in Animal Husbandry and Veterinary Medicine, chaired by Michael Meredith Swann (1920–1990), a distinguished molecular and cell biologist and principal and vice chancellor of Edinburgh University.

The Swann Committee obtained evidence from expert witnesses and selected publications. In 1967 most antibiotics, approximately 240 tons, were used in humans, whereas 168 tons were used in animals (approximately 88 tons of which were used in animal feed).[10] The practice of administering antibiotics to livestock was divided into three categories: growth promotion (used solely to promote growth), therapy (used to treat sick animals), and prophylaxis (used to prevent infection in stressed animals).

The use of antibiotics as growth promoters was distinct from therapeutic use; levels as low as 1 to 2 parts per million produced significant responses in animal growth. Much higher doses of antibiotics, up to 100 parts per million or more, were used to treat sick animals. The veterinary community believed that the higher doses needed to treat sick animals promoted antibiotic resistance, not the minute levels used for growth promotion.[11]

By one account, committee members recognized the importance of antibiotics used in the first two categories, growth promotion and treatment, but considered the third category, disease prevention, less important.[12] The committee defined "stress" as an adverse reaction in an animal that had encountered an environmental change. "Stressed" animals were considered to be more vulnerable to infections and likely to benefit from antibiotic prophylaxis.[13] The committee discussed microbial risks. Enteric (gut) bacteria generated the most discussion. Of these, the salmonellas were the main disease-causing microbes of concern, largely because of the *Salmonella typhimurium* type 29 outbreak that had peaked in 1965.[14]

The Swann Report, issued in November 1969, concluded that administering antibiotics to livestock for growth promotion and other purposes posed hazards to human and animal health by promoting antibiotic-resistant strains in enteric bacteria of animal origin. The resistant strains were found to transmit resistance factors to other bacteria, posing serious threats if highly lethal organisms such as *Salmonella typhi* (the causative agent of typhoid fever) were to acquire such capabilities. However, the committee recognized the important role that low concentrations of antibiotics played in the growth rates of young pigs and poultry; this practice had commercial advantages. The committee recommended that antibiotics of considerable importance as therapeutics in humans or animals not be used as "feed" antibiotics. Therefore, chlortetracycline, oxytetracycline, penicillin, tylosin, sulfonamides, and nitrofuran drugs should be available only by prescription for therapeutic purposes. Chloramphenicol, a powerful antibiotic not widely used in human medicine because of its risk of causing a potentially fatal blood disease, should be reserved for special situations. Feed antibiotics should be available without prescription for pigs and poultry as well as for calves up to three months of age. For sick animals, veterinarians should have no limit to the number and types of antibiotics available to use. The committee recommended that alternative methods of growth promotion be investigated, that human and veterinary epidemiological surveillance of bacterial resistance be continued, and that one committee should have overall responsibility for the oversight of antibiotic use in humans and animals and for other purposes.[15]

The farming and pharmaceutical industries voiced strong opposition to the Swann Report's recommendations. They believed that the recommendations were based on scanty scientific evidence and demanded more research.[16] They asserted that the outbreak of *S. typhimurium* type 29 in calves was the result of poor animal-husbandry practices rather than the administration of antibiotics.[17] According to one report, Cyanamid, a pharmaceutical company, hired a public relations firm to collect more than 100 press and journal articles antagonistic to the recommendations, focusing on the increased costs to the industry and the likely increased costs passed on to consumers.[18]

Despite opposition, on November 20, 1969, Cledwyn Hughes, the minister of MAFF, presented the Swann Report's findings and recommendations to the British House of Commons, stating that in general, MAFF accepted the committee's recommendations to control antibiotics, but that some of the recommendations and long-term proposals needed further study. Some members of the House of Commons expressed concerns about the adverse impact on animal husbandry and the potential increased food-production costs if the recommendations were implemented. One member wondered if the livestock industry itself might voluntarily stop adding antibiotics to feedstuffs.[19]

The House of Commons proposed banning three antibiotic feed additives: chlortetracycline, oxytetracycline, and penicillin. In agreement with the Swann recommendations, a distinction would be made between feed and therapeutic antibiotics: feed antibiotics would be available without a prescription;

therapeutic antibiotics would be available only by prescription from a veterinary practitioner. Richard Crossman (1907–1974), the secretary of state for Health and Social Security, said that the expected ban would take place over several months, not weeks or years. This would allow the present stocks of feed additives to be depleted, as the matter was not believed to be so urgent as to cause unnecessary panic or economic loss.[20]

While the Labour government accepted the Swann Report's recommendations in 1969, it was the Conservative government elected in 1970 that passed it under the Medicines Act. By then, the *S. typhimurium* type 29 epidemic in calves had abated, for reasons not completely understood; however, the practice of selling and sending very young calves on long journeys with antibiotics slung around their necks in case they developed diarrhea proved to be unprofitable, and tetracycline was no longer widely used as a growth promoter.[21]

There are conflicting reports as to exactly when the government implemented the Swann Report recommendations. One account stated that they were implemented in 1971.[22] Another said that at least one recommendation, the formation of a powerful committee to oversee the use of antibiotics in humans and livestock, was not implemented until 1973. Unfortunately, the committee that the ministers formed, the Joint Sub-Committee on Antimicrobial Substances (JCAMS), a combination of the Committee for Safety of Medicines of the Department of Health and Social Security and the Veterinary Products Committee of MAFF, had neither the power nor the resources to do its job. As a subcommittee, JCAMS could advise but not make decisions. It could not obtain information from the pharmaceutical industry about the amount of antibiotics used in humans and animals. It could not review the subsequent impact of approved antibiotics. It was unable to secure resources to conduct field studies and laboratory investigations to monitor antibiotic resistance. It was unable to stop companies from advertising antibiotics in farming journals and encouraging farmers and veterinarians to use their products, despite evidence of overuse and resistance. Frustrated, the subcommittee members developed detailed proposals for their subcommittee's reform, with increased oversight powers, and submitted them to the ministers of Health and Agriculture. In response, in 1981 the ministers disbanded the group.[23]

Unfortunately, as the British government rolled back the implementation of the Swann Report's recommendations, outbreaks of new multi-drug-resistant strains of *S. typhimurium* types 204 and 193 were appearing in bovines and humans throughout the United Kingdom. An editorial in the *British Medical Journal* speculated as to why the legislation to enact the Swann Report's recommendations had failed to prevent the development of new multi-drug-resistant organisms in animals and humans. By late 1979, more than 300 cases of human salmonellosis had appeared, including two deaths involving two resistant strains. The cases were not confined to farming families. Some blamed the veterinary profession, but others highlighted the role of the medical profession in readily prescribing antibiotics.[24]

In early October 1981, the Association of Veterinarians in Industries held a symposium to assess what progress, if any, had been made since the Swann Report. Sir James Howie (1907–1995), professor of immunology at the University of Glasgow, noted that it was ironic that new types of multiple-resistant salmonellas were occurring 10 years later because the Swann Report's recommendations had been poorly implemented or, in some cases, not implemented at all. Sir Howie mentioned that in the early 1970s there had been a joint British Medical Association–British Veterinary Medical Association Committee. He believed that it should be reconvened to address the serious matter of antimicrobial resistance and that the Swann Report's recommendations needed to be reexamined, updated, and implemented.[25]

According to Dr. E. John Threlfall, former director of the Laboratory of Enteric Pathogens, Centre for Infections, UK Health Protection Agency, the Swann Report's recommendations, resulting in the ban on the use of some antibiotics as growth promoters in livestock, did not have much impact on the use of antibiotics for therapy or prophylaxis. Antibiotics that had previously been used for growth promotion were subsequently being used for prophylaxis; the end result was an increase in usage.[26]

Since 1993, the Veterinary Medicines Directorate of the Ministry of Agriculture, Fisheries and Food, subsequently renamed the Department for the Environment, Food, and Rural Affairs (DEFRA), has monitored the sales of veterinary antimicrobial products in the United Kingdom. Total antimicrobial sales in livestock peaked in 1996 to approximately 533 tons of active ingredient.[27]

Sales of growth-promoting antibiotics peaked in 1998 before dropping to zero in 2006 as a result of the EU ban.[28] After the ban, total antibiotic sales atypically peaked in 2010 at 390 tons, dropped 100 tons in 2011, then settled back to approximately 2009 levels.[29] These fluctuations were attributed to consumer responses to changes in the corporations that sold the products.[30]

Nevertheless, from 1998 to 2013, therapeutic antibiotic use increased 41 percent, but total overall antibiotic use decreased approximately 10 percent, since growth-promoting antibiotics were no longer used.*

However, although antibiotic growth-promoting use ceased, poultry farmers still needed something to prevent coccidiosis and necrotic enteritis in their flocks.[31] Use of coccidiostats, antiparasitic agents that control against these diseases in poultry, increased 45 percent after the 2006 ban. But the long-term trend since 1998 showed a threefold increase in use.[32] Coccidiostats are not used in human medicine.*

From 1998 to 2013, tetracyclines were the most commonly used antibiotics in livestock, and products for pigs and poultry constituted the largest tonnage of active ingredients sold. Pigs used 61 tons of antibiotics in 2013, and poultry used 19 tons. Products targeted for both species together sold 226 tons in 2013—a 5 percent decline from 1998.*[33] Human antibiotic sales data appears in chapter 6.

Despite the United Kingdom's ban of several growth-promoting antibiotics, problems with *Salmonella* continued. By the early 1980s, a new multi-resistant strain of *S. typhimurium* appeared—definitive phage type (DT) 104. In 1989 the strain became epidemic in cattle. Unlike previous resistant *S. typhimurium* strains, which were found primarily in cattle, DT 104 spread to pigs, poultry, and sheep. People became infected by eating beef, pork sausages, chicken, and meat paste as well as by close contact with infected cattle. The DT 104 epidemic prompted MAFF to fund a study examining the possible sources of the cattle herds' infection. The study found that wild birds and cats were associated with an increased risk of the disease, especially if they had access to the cattle-feed stores. Cats were found to carry the multi-drug-resistant pathogen. Other risk factors included herd calving time, close confinement of cattle in buildings, lack of isolation facilities for sick cattle, and newly purchased potentially infectious cattle.[34]

Alison Mather and colleagues at the University of Glasgow and the University of Guelph, Ontario, Canada, used a population-biology approach, combining ecology and epidemiology, to research the problem of resistant *S. typhimurium* DT 104 in Scotland. One of their goals was to determine whether the resistant microbes in livestock, primarily cattle, and in humans came from a common ancestor or whether they constituted two separate populations. Using 5,200 human and livestock DT 104 specimens submitted to the Scottish *Salmonella, Shigella,* and *Clostridium difficile* Reference Laboratory over a 15-year period

(1990 to 2004), they developed mathematical models and conducted numerous statistical tests. Their results indicated that the human cases of resistant *S. typhimurium* DT 104 were unlikely to have originated in the livestock population in Scotland; the human and animal microbial communities appeared separate and distinguishable. Most of the resistant DT 104 populations common to both humans and animals were first identified in humans. They recommended that imported food should be examined as a possible source of human infection.[35]

The study was criticized. Peter Collingnon, an infectious-disease specialist in Australia, believed the methodologies were limited and the conclusions misleading. He thought the authors had neglected to acknowledge the decades worth of data demonstrating the link between antibiotic use in livestock and subsequent human illnesses and deaths. Even worse, he indicated, their study provided ammunition for some groups to defend the use of antibiotics on farms.[36]

The authors of the Scottish study defended their work, stating that their focus was on animal populations—not just animal production. They believed their methodology was sound and pointed out that their conclusions applied only to Scotland. They did agree with the critics, however, that antimicrobial resistance is one of the greatest challenges facing human and animal health.[37]

The British Veterinary Medical Association's (BVA's) website welcomed the research findings from the University of Glasgow, indicating that antibiotic use in livestock posed a lower risk to humans than previously thought. The website stated that the research should call into question the European Parliament's policies to ban the prophylactic use of antibiotics in livestock. Carl Padgett, the president of the BVA, stated that antimicrobial resistance in humans had been blamed on the veterinary use of antibiotics, restricting veterinarians' ability to use certain classes of these drugs.[38]

In June 2011 the *Independent,* one of Britain's newest national morning newspapers, published an article titled "Death Wish: Routine Use of Vital Antibiotics on Farms Threatens Human Health." The article stated that three antibiotics, cephalosporins, fluoroquinolones, and macrolides, all important medical therapeutics, had increased in use up to eightfold over the previous decade in animal populations. British scientists had identified a new type of methicillin-resistant *Staphylococcus aureus* in milk—a first. This development was blamed on the use of antibiotics in dairy cows to prevent mastitis, an infection of the udder. Mastitis occurs more frequently in cows that are milked intensively. The Soil Association demanded an end to routine antibiotic use in dairy farming.[39]

On its Antibiotic Resistance web page, the National Office of Animal Health, an organization representing the UK animal-medicine industry, stated that antimicrobial resistance in animals could be transmitted (to humans) indirectly via organisms such as enterococcus or *E. coli* that normally reside in guts, but the problem is primarily one of poor hygienic practices in food preparation rather than antibiotic use in animals. Veterinary medicines, including antimicrobials, were necessary to ensure healthy animals in the United Kingdom. The website also said that although antibiotic resistance is a serious issue in chronic conditions, such as methicillin-resistant *S. aureus* and tuberculosis, and in some hospital settings, it is rarely an issue in animals.[40]

The United Kingdom was one of the first nations to investigate the problem of antimicrobial resistance in humans and livestock; the Swann Report made important recommendations that the British Parliament partially enacted. But British farmers and the pharmaceutical industry were largely opposed to any changes in livestock production. Without their cooperation and support, implementing changes in antibiotic use would be difficult. Antibiotic sales data for livestock before and after the 2006 ban suggests that overall use declined minimally.

Evaluating the ban's impact on resistant *S. typhimurium* is difficult because the organism has a broad range of hosts besides livestock, including cats, dogs, rodents, hedgehogs, birds, reptiles, amphibians, and fish. These animals could serve as additional sources of resistant *Salmonella*. For example, an outbreak of tetracycline-resistant *S. typhimurium* occurred in 2008 in England and Wales. It was caused by mice shipped from the United States to feed pet reptiles.[41] Reducing resistant *S. typhimurium* infections requires extensive surveillance and control efforts. Sweden is one country that has been successful in reducing *S. typhimurium* in its livestock; its experience with banning antibiotic growth-promoting agents is explored in the next chapter.

CHAPTER FOUR

Lessons from Sweden

In 1986 Sweden became the first country to completely ban the use of antibiotic growth promoters in animal feed. The Swedish debate on the use of antibiotics in animal feed was intertwined with concerns about the environment and animal welfare. The publication of *Silent Spring* in 1962 prompted a long-standing interest in environmental protection.[1]

Swedish veterinarians were among the first professional groups that voiced concerns about agriculture's growing dependence on automation, pesticides, liquid manure systems, and antibiotics, believing that these developments jeopardized animal health and welfare. They were concerned that antibiotics covered up poor farm hygiene and management practices and took the Swann Report's recommendations seriously. In 1977 the Swedish government implemented some of the Swann Report's recommendations by banning from use in animal feeds certain antibiotics that were important for human health. Unlike other countries, Sweden prohibited veterinarians from selling drugs directly to consumers, such as farmers, thereby eliminating a potential conflict of interest. Instead, the National Corporation of Pharmacies maintained strict control of antibiotic sales.[2]

A series of newspaper articles published in 1981 in *Dagens Nyheter* (Daily news), Sweden's largest daily paper, brought public awareness to new heights regarding the use of low-dose antibiotics in animal feed. One article reported that more than 30 tons of low-dose antibiotic feed additives were given to livestock each year.[3] The public was outraged that antibiotics were fed to healthy animals and strongly criticized the practice. A public debate ensued, and officials working for Swedish farming organizations took notice.[4]

Gunnela Stahle, an agronomist with the Federation of Swedish Farmers, recalled what happened:

Gunilla Krantz, a former information officer with the Swedish Dairy Association, working for the Swedish farmer-owned Meat Marketing Association, suggested to me that the Federation of Swedish Farmers (LRF) should respond to
the public criticism of using antibiotics in animal feed. At that time, I was responsible for food safety and animal welfare at LRF. My boss, the president of
the Swedish Farmers and the board, was supportive of the idea of banning antibiotic growth promoters. LRF made a request to the competent authorities for a
ban, but the request was rejected in 1983, claiming that a ban was not necessary
for safety reasons.[5]

Stahle and like-minded colleagues worked behind the scenes to generate support for a ban. In 1984 the LRF general assembly reached consensus on the
issue and subsequently petitioned the government to ban antibiotic growth
promoters. Some members of the Swedish Parliament presented motions also
asking for a ban. In 1985 Parliament passed the Feedingstuffs Act, which included the ban. The farmers wanted a legal mandate, not a voluntary ban,
because they knew that a voluntary ban would not be as effective. Their main
argument for the ban was to build consumer confidence in Swedish meat and
to reduce antimicrobial resistance.[6] Ultimately, they wanted to have the
"cleanest agriculture in the world."[7]

Impact from the Antibiotic Growth Promoter Ban

The farmers most affected by the ban were the broiler poultry (chickens raised
for meat) and pig producers, who relied on antibiotics to promote growth and
prevent disease. They wanted compensation from the Swedish government
to cover their expenses for changing their livestock production methods to
exclude antibiotic growth promoters. They got the ban, the 1986 Feedingstuffs Act, but not the compensation. Antibiotics would be allowed only with
a veterinarian's prescription for preventive and therapeutic purposes.[8]

Two years after the Feedingstuffs Act, the Swedish Parliament passed stricter
rules for animal protection and welfare, including new space requirements for
livestock, a maximum weaning age of four weeks for pigs, and the require-
ment to use straw or litter for pig stalls. These rules, fully in effect since 1994,
together with the ban on antibiotic growth promoters, transformed Swedish
livestock production, making it more humane and ecologically sustainable.[9]
Most importantly, the farmers supported and adhered to them.

National sales data showed that the ban was highly effective in curtailing antibiotic use in livestock. In 1980, six years before the ban, 8,380 kilograms of active antibiotic substances were sold as feed additives; in 1984 sales had decreased to 700 kilograms. By 1988, two years after the ban, total sales for feed additives dropped to zero.[10] In addition, total sales of antibiotics decreased 76 percent from 1984 (50 tons) to 2012 (11.7 tons).*[11]

Broiler poultry farmers had a long history of relying on antibiotics and were given an additional two years beyond the ban's January 1, 1986, deadline to curtail their use of antibacterial feed additives.[12] Nitrovin, an antibiotic given to broiler chickens in the 1970s, was highly successful at eliminating necrotic enteritis. Nitrovin was replaced by avoparcin, an antibiotic chemically similar to vancomycin, an important human therapeutic agent. In the early 1980s, Sweden stopped using avoparcin because studies suggested that it made poultry more susceptible to *Salmonella*.[13]

Sweden worked hard to control *Salmonella* through its decades-long, stringent *Salmonella* control program; as a result, the prevalence of the bacteria in live animals and animal products was very low.[14] The country did not want to jeopardize its hard-earned success by using avoparcin.[15] The decision to replace avoparcin with virginiamycin was fortuitous, because about a decade later, avoparcin was found to be associated with vancomycin-resistant enterococci (VRE), a deadly disease in humans.[16] VRE is discussed further in chapters 5, 6, and 7.

However, broiler producers still needed pharmacological assistance against coccidiosis, a deadly parasitic infection, and necrotic enteritis, a severe intestinal disorder resulting from *Clostridium perfringens*.[17] Government officials decided that coccidiostats would be exempted from the ban indefinitely.[18] From 1984 to 2011, sales of coccidiostats increased 86 percent.*[19] In addition to using coccidiostats, the poultry industry needed to make changes in feed composition such as adding enzymes and probiotics and reducing proteins. It also needed to improve farm hygiene to promote weight gain and prevent disease.[20]

However, many believed that the ban was implemented too quickly. During the first year, 90 percent of the broiler chickens required continuous treatment with virginiamycin at a dose of 20 ppm (double the typical growth-promoter dose); one year later, 100 percent of the chickens had to be treated. Virginiamycin was gradually replaced by a two-day course of phenoxy methyl penicillin in drinking water during outbreaks of necrotic enteritis. This treatment, too, was subsequently replaced by the occasional use of tylosin, another antibiotic. Since 1995, outbreaks of necrotic enteritis rarely occur.[21]

Pig farmers, especially those raising piglets, had more difficulty with the ban than the poultry farmers. Weaning piglets (pigs weighing less than 20 kilograms, or approximately 44 pounds) is often wrought with challenges. Multiple factors, including age, stress, hygiene, and feed composition, affect piglet weaning. Weaning piglets left alone without their sow (mother) become stressed and require strategies such as keeping litters together and providing tasty feed to promote their growth and well-being. Piglets are also prone to developing scours (severe diarrhea). Zinc oxide, a nonantibiotic feed additive, helps prevent scours and promotes growth.[22] Since 1992 it has been allowed in piglet production at 2,000 ppm, but only with a prescription from a veterinarian.[23] Use of zinc oxide in Sweden increased 631 percent from 2000 to 2008.* Data after 2008 is not available. Unfortunately, excessive amounts of zinc in animal manure from intensive pig farming can accumulate in the topsoil, potentially causing toxicity to microorganisms and plants and adversely affecting environmental health.[24]

Some farmers implemented the needed changes in animal and farm hygiene and management more readily than others. Some veterinarians were lax in prescribing antibiotics, while others were strict. The absence of antibiotics in feed negatively affected livestock production and increased animal disease and mortality. In 1997 the Swedish Farmers Feed Development, the Swedish Meat Marketing Association, and Swedish pig producers authorized the Swedish University of Agriculture to conduct a study analyzing the costs versus benefits of the 1986 Feedingstuffs Act and the 1988 Animal Welfare law. The study concluded that the increased production costs were offset by the improvements in animal health, improved feed conversion, and increased daily weight gain.[25]

From 1981 to 1993, Swedish broiler chicken production and consumption increased 62 percent; importation of broiler meat was minimal until 1990, averaging less than 2 million kg per year. Over the next 18 years, from 1994 to 2012, Swedish broiler production increased 56 percent, but not as much as consumption, which increased approximately 150 percent. Swedish broiler production could not meet consumer demands, so broiler imports increased thirty-eight-fold after Sweden joined the European Union in 1995. In 2012 almost 180 tons of broiler meat were imported.* [26]

Broiler production became more efficient through increased farm sizes, but the price for domestic poultry meat remained higher than that for imported meat. Many Swedish consumers were willing to pay higher prices for fresh domestically produced meat to benefit animal welfare, but frozen products faced stiffer competition from the cheaper imports. Although fresh meat sold in retail stores was domestically produced, poultry meat consumed in restaurants was almost always imported. Over the years, eating in restaurants became increasingly popular.[27]

Countries such as Thailand have lower poultry production costs and send many of their products to the European Union, but the Swedish Board of Agriculture records only the last country before entry, which is typically Denmark.[28] In the first six months of 2013, 44 percent of the salted or prepared imported poultry meat came from Denmark, 15 percent from Thailand, 12 percent from the Netherlands, and 11 percent from Germany.[29]

From 1982 to 2012, the consumer price index (CPI) for broilers rose 25 percent. Increased efficiency in domestic broiler production and competition from cheaper imports were likely two important reasons why the CPI for broilers was flatter than that for pork, which increased 82 percent.*[30]

Pig farming changed, too. From 1980 to 1990, before Sweden joined the European Union, the number of pig farms decreased by more than 50 percent.*[31] Like the poultry farmers, some pig producers increased their herd size to hundreds of animals; others went out of business.[32] From 1980 to 2012, the total number of pigs in the country decreased almost 50 percent, and the number of pigs slaughtered at slaughterhouses decreased 38 percent.[33]

As with broiler production, Swedish pork production could not meet consumer demand.[34] As a result, from 1994 to 2012, Sweden's importation of pork increased ninefold. Most of the imported pork came from Denmark and Germany.* Gunnela Stahle, expert with the Swedish Farmers, attributed most of the decrease in Swedish pork production to increased competition from imported meat after Sweden joined the European Union. Swedish consumers preferred Swedish meat and paid more for it, but the higher prices did not benefit the farmers. Many Swedish pig farmers went out of business because of lack of profitability.[35]

Antibiotic Resistance Monitoring

In 2000 and 2001, the Swedish National Veterinary Institute and the Swedish Institute for Communicable Disease Control began publishing annual data on antimicrobial resistance in animals and humans, respectively.[36] The Swedish Veterinary Antimicrobial Resistance Monitoring (SVARM) reports divided bacteria into three categories: zoonotic, indicator, and animal pathogens. *Salmonella* and *Campylobacter* (*Campylobacter jejuni* and *Campylobacter coli*) species were categorized as zoonotic bacteria because they reside in the guts of poultry and many other animals, potentially causing disease in both animals and humans. They can also develop antimicrobial resistance. Indicator bacteria, such as *Escherichia coli* and *Enterococcus,* normally reside in healthy animal and human intestines, but they can cause disease and acquire resistance genes and transfer them to other bacterial species.[37] Animal pathogens cause diseases only in animals, not in humans; therefore, they are not discussed here.

Resistance rates for *Salmonella typhimurium, Campylobacter,* and *E. coli* in animals were available in the 2000–2012 SVARM reports. Antimicrobial resistance rates in humans were published in the 2001–11 Swedish Antibiotic Utilization and Resistance in Human Medicine (SWEDRES) reports.[38] Unfortunately, minimal SVARM or SWEDRES antimicrobial resistance data was available before Sweden's antibiotic growth promoter ban, making before-and-after-ban comparisons difficult.

The only preban SVARM antibiotic resistance data available was for *S. typhimurium,* showing that from 1978 to 1988, 74 percent of the 125 *S. typhimurium* isolates tested were resistant to streptomycin; 13 percent were resistant to tetracycline. These early isolates were from cattle.[39] After the ban, from 1989 to 2012, a total of 997 *S. typhimurium* isolates were collected from animals (an average of 45 specimens per year).[40] Approximately half of the isolates were from livestock.[41] The other half were from dogs, cats, horses, and wildlife. Resistance to streptomycin plummeted from 74 percent to 15 percent around the time of the ban and never regained preban levels; reasons for the decrease are unclear. Streptomycin was not listed as a growth-promoting agent in the SVARM 2000 report.[42] Resistance rates to streptomycin fluctuated, reaching levels as high as 27 percent in 2012. Similarly, sulfonamide, ampicillin, and tetracycline resistance rates fluctuated, reaching, in 2012, peak levels of 20 percent, 16 percent, and 14 percent, respectively.*[43]

The Swedish *Salmonella* control program screened and eliminated contaminated feedstuffs and animals. It was established long before the 1986 antibiotic ban.[44] This program's success meant that most cases of human salmonellosis occurred in Swedes traveling abroad or consuming imported food products.

Fluoroquinolones were commonly used in human medicine in Sweden, but minimally in livestock.[45] From 1978 to 2011 the *S. typhimurium* resistance rate against ciprofloxacin in domestic and wild animals has been zero, with two exceptions: 2008 (3%) and 2009 (1%).[46]

In 2012 Sweden sold more antibiotics for systemic and intestinal anti-infective treatment in humans than in animals:[47] 64.9 tons versus 11.6 tons, respectively. Except for aminoglycosides (e.g., streptomycin) and trimethoprim-sulfonamides, human use of antibiotics far exceeded veterinary use.[48] Beta-lactamase-sensitive penicillins and tetracyclines were the two most commonly used antibiotics in people.[49] The highest antibiotic sales for veterinary use were for penicillin, sulfonamides, and tetracyclines. With the exception of tetracyclines, these antibiotics were primarily used to treat individual sick animals.[50] Tetracyclines and macrolides/lincosamides (e.g., erythromycin and clindamycin) were mostly used to treat groups of animals (i.e., herds and flocks).[51]

The Swedish experience of banning antibiotic growth-promoting agents illustrates the complexity of the interactions between humans and animals. Unfortunately, the ban's impact on antimicrobial resistance in humans is indeterminate. Most of Sweden's data on antimicrobial resistance in humans and animals covers only the postban years, with the exception of data on *S. typhimurium*.

While Sweden does not have enough data to make before- and after-ban comparisons, Denmark does, particularly regarding the rise of vancomycin-resistant *Enterococcus faecium* (VRE) as a result of avoparcin use. Denmark banned avoparcin and subsequently all growth-promoting antibiotics. Its pre- and postban experience will examined in chapter 5.

CHAPTER FIVE

Lessons from Denmark

Vancomycin had been used for many years against *Enterococcus faecium* without resistance developing, leading many in the medical community to assume that resistance would never appear. Unfortunately, that assumption proved to be wrong. In 1988 there were case reports of vancomycin-resistant *E. faecium* (VRE) in seriously ill patients in Paris and London.[1] They were the first human cases of VRE reported.[2] In Paris, patients with fever and neutropenia (low white blood cell counts) had been receiving vancomycin and other antibiotics as empiric treatment. Similarly, in London, three months before the VRE outbreak, a new policy had been adopted: administer vancomycin and ceftazidime (a third-generation cephalosporin) to all patients with fever and undiagnosed infections. No proven therapy for VRE existed.[3]

A few years later, VRE was isolated from food animals in England and Germany.[4] Avoparcin, a growth-promoting antibiotic chemically related to vancomycin was implicated as the cause.[5] The use of avoparcin in livestock and the finding of VRE in frozen poultry, raw minced pig meat, and fecal samples from 12 out of 100 healthy humans living in rural areas led to the conclusion that farm animals were important reservoirs of VRE.[6] This finding generated worldwide concern.

Infections from enterococci (i.e., *E. faecium* and *Enterococcus faecalis*) can be fatal. Treatment typically involved penicillin (e.g., ampicillin) plus an aminoglycoside (e.g., gentamicin).[7] However, high rates of ampicillin resistance have led to more potent therapies such as vancomycin, linezolid, or quinupristin-dalfopristin.[8] Only vancomycin is effective against both *E. faecium* and *E. faecalis*, but unfortunately, rising rates of vancomycin resistance have been undermining its usefulness. Linezolid and quinupristin-dalfopristin are effective only against *E. faecium*.*[9]

The Danish Experience

At the Danish Veterinary Association's annual meeting in 1994, scientists were concerned about the general use of antibiotics in livestock. Increasing tetracycline use in livestock resulted in a rise in tetracycline resistance in bacteria isolated from their feces. A heated debate ensued over veterinarians earning enormous profits from selling antibiotics to farmers who used these drugs primarily for growth promotion.[10]

Frank Aarestrup, a graduate student at the time, working on his PhD in bovine mastitis, recalled what happened:

> The debate was not really about science, but more about the ethics and whether vets should make a living from selling drugs or ensuring that animals are healthy. The debate did not end, but eventually was stopped, and everybody went out to drink beer. A journalist subsequently profiled the story on TV, and everybody from the minister to the farmers could see that using tetracycline as top dressing was not really responsible. So everybody agreed that something needed to be done. Thus, the interventions.[11]

On January 25, 1995, Danish scientists identified VRE while screening fecal samples from healthy chickens and pigs. Denmark relied heavily on growth-promoting antibiotics, including avoparcin.*[12] This finding led to considerable scientific and public concern. Officials at the Pig Research Centre, Danish Agriculture and Food Council, declared that animal management practices had to change:

> Antibiotic growth promoter use in pigs was increasing in the 1990s, but the effect of avoparcin on vancomycin resistance prompted us to rethink what we were doing. Some of the companies producing growth-promoting antibiotics doubted the findings, but clearly the practice was no longer acceptable. Everyone agreed that antibiotics should only be used when animals were sick. Since the 1800s, all Danish pig-producing entities have been owned by the pig farmers themselves from the field, to the slaughterhouse, to the processing companies. After a series of meetings, we reached an agreement with the feedstock companies that they wouldn't add growth-promoting antibiotics anymore to the animal feed. And pig farmers agreed that they would no longer deliver pigs raised on antibiotics to slaughterhouses. This agreement was more or less voluntary, but the farmers would be punished if they didn't comply. But without a

doubt, producing pigs is much more difficult without growth-promoting anti-biotics than with them. Much higher standards of animal management are required.[13]

The Danish Growth-Promoter Ban

Although the Danish pig farmers voluntarily stopped using avoparcin for growth promotion in May 1995, the Danish Ministry of Agriculture and Fish-eries went a step further and banned its use in an effort to preserve the clinical effectiveness of vancomycin. The ban was controversial and not supported by the EU Scientific Committee on Animal Nutrition; however, the European Council of Ministers upheld it. One year later, Germany banned avoparcin use as well. In 1997 all European Union member states banned avoparcin.[14]

Concerns about antimicrobial resistance prompted the Danish Ministry of Health and the Danish Ministry of Food, Agriculture, and Fisheries to jointly launch a national surveillance and research program, the Danish Integrated Antimicrobial Resistance Monitoring and Research Program (DANMAP), to monitor bacterial resistance in animals, food, and humans. The Danish Vet-erinary Laboratory, the National Food Agency of Denmark, and the Statens Serum Institut collaborated in producing the first DANMAP report in Febru-ary 1997. Since then, DANMAP reports have been issued annually.[15]

From 1990 to 1994, Denmark increased its annual total consumption of antibiotics in livestock, which peaked in 1994 at almost 116,000 kilograms of active substance, primarily in pigs, just before the voluntary ban on growth-promoting antibiotics commenced.*[16] Avoparcin accounted for more than 20 percent of the antibiotics. In 1995 pigs received 86 percent of the growth-promoting antibiotics, cattle 7 percent, and broilers 5 percent.[17] Therefore, the ban on growth-promoting antibiotics affected primarily pig farming, similar to what happened in the United Kingdom and Sweden.[18]

In January 1998 the Danish authorities banned the growth-promoting an-tibiotic virginiamycin,[19] which is related to the antibiotics quinupristin and dalfopristin, medications used jointly to treat vancomycin-resistant *E. faecium*. One month later, in response to consumer concerns, the Danish cattle and broiler poultry industries voluntarily stopped using *all* antimicrobial growth promoters, and the pig industry voluntarily stopped using antimicrobial growth promoters in "finishing" pigs (pigs weighing more than 35 kg [77 lbs.]). A little more than a year later, the pig industry voluntarily stopped using anti-biotic growth promoters in all pigs.[20]

The goal of Denmark's ban on antibiotic growth promoters was to reduce the emergence and spread of antibiotic-resistant bacteria, particularly enterococci, without adversely impacting livestock production. To evaluate the impact of the ban, the World Health Organization convened a panel of independent interdisciplinary experts in November 2002, three years after the use of growth-promoting antibiotics ceased.[21] The experts noted that the antimicrobial growth promoters used in Denmark were active primarily against Gram-positive bacteria, such as *E. faecium* and *E. faecalis,* so effects of their termination on Gram-negative bacteria, such as *Salmonella, Campylobacter,* and *Escherichia coli,* would not be expected.[22] Therefore, the analysis in this chapter focuses primarily on *E. faecium,* since it has demonstrated higher resistance rates than *E. faecalis.*

Unfortunately, the ban on growth-promoting agents led to an increase in postweaning diarrhea in pigs, necessitating the increased use of tetracycline. DANMAP data from 1998 to 2010 showed an almost 120 percent increase in the use of therapeutic antibiotics, primarily tetracyclines but also beta-lactamase-sensitive penicillins and macrolides (e.g., erythromycin), plus lincosamides (e.g., streptomycin), mostly in pigs.*[23] Concerned by the dramatic increase in therapeutic antibiotic use, the Danish Veterinary and Food Administration (DVFA) implemented a "yellow card" initiative in 2010, targeting pig producers. The DVFA's goal was to reduce therapeutic antibiotic usage by 10 percent by setting threshold limits of average antimicrobial consumption over nine-month periods. If the threshold limits were exceeded, then orders or injunctions (i.e., yellow cards) were issued, requiring the farmer to pay a fee for each injunction, all inspection visits, and other expenses, including expert veterinarian advice.[24] The yellow-card initiative successfully reduced antibiotic usage by 20 percent in 2012, but by 2013 use slightly increased again.[25] Antibiotic use in livestock, primarily pigs, still far surpassed use in clinical medicine.*[26] In 2014 Denmark announced plans to reduce antibiotic use in pigs by half by 2015.[27]

The increase in tetracycline use after 1997 led to a more than 4.4-fold increase in resistant *Salmonella typhimurium* in pigs. In humans, *S. typhimurium* gastrointestinal infections acquired domestically showed a dramatic drop in tetracycline resistance in 2009 but then rebounded in subsequent years, ultimately resulting in an almost threefold increase in resistance compared to 1997.*[28] The resistance rates between pigs and humans were highly correlated (R = 0.60; fig. 5.1).

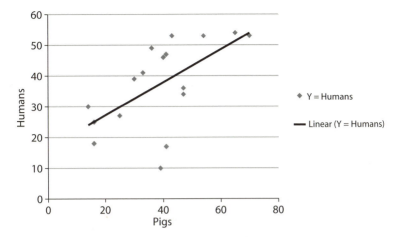

Fig. 5.1. Correlation between pigs and human domestically acquired infections: *Salmonella typhimurium* tetracycline resistance. Correlation = 0.60. *Source:* Based on DANMAP data.

Despite the increase in *Salmonella* tetracycline resistance, WHO experts concluded that the ban was successful because it led to a decline in antibiotic-resistant enterococci in livestock. (Most enteric nontyphoidal *Salmonella* infections resolve without antibiotics in immune-intact individuals;[29] serious infections require treatment with third-generation cephalosporins or fluoroquinolones, not tetracycline.)[30]

E. faecium isolates from slaughtered chickens and pigs showed reduced resistance to growth-promoting antibiotics such as streptogramins, avilamycin, and avoparcin.[31] And they showed reduced resistance to antibiotics used in clinical medicine. For example, from 1997 to 2002, *E. faecium* resistance to erythromycin decreased 82 percent in broiler chickens and 72 percent in pigs, but the trend reversed temporarily in 2003. In humans, erythromycin resistance increased threefold from 2002 to 2006,[32] correlating highly with the temporarily increased resistance rate in pigs.*

The increase in erythromycin resistance was likely due to tylosin, a macrolide antibiotic similar to erythromycin, which was used as both a growth-promoting and a therapeutic agent in pigs.[33] Enterococci resistance to erythromycin declined when tylosin use decreased. WHO experts believed that tylosin had a greater impact on erythromycin resistance when used as a growth-promoting agent than when used as a therapeutic agent. Their conclusion was based on industry statements regarding tylosin use in weaner versus finisher pigs. Finisher pigs were bigger than the younger, weaner pigs and ate more feed laced with growth-promoting antibiotics.[34]

The avoparcin ban had a tremendous impact on *E. faecium* vancomycin resistance cultured from livestock. From 1997 to 2007, this organism underwent a 90 percent reduction in vancomycin resistance in broilers and pigs.*[35] But VRE did not completely disappear from livestock. Fifteen years after the ban, VRE was detected in Danish broilers. Reasons for this are unknown. No change was observed for *E. faecalis,* since its resistance to vancomycin was zero virtually every year.[36]

Unfortunately, no data on healthy humans before the avoparcin ban is available. In 2002 Denmark began a screening program of healthy volunteers randomly selected from the Danish Civil Register System, which included all residents in Denmark.[37] Virtually all enterococci specimens from these volunteers had zero resistance to vancomycin.

There was one notable exception. Sometime between 2002 and 2003, approximately seven years after the ban, VRE was isolated from a healthy female volunteer. Genetic analysis of the resistant organism revealed pig origin, raising concerns that coselection effects from the therapeutic use of tetracycline in pigs could have been responsible for the finding. (Many *E. faecium* isolates resistant to tetracycline were also resistant to vancomycin.)[38] Another possible explanation was the continued use of tylosin, since resistance genes for vancomycin and for tylosin were located on the same plasmid.[39] The gene encoding for vancomycin resistance has been shown to be transferable between bacteria inside the human intestine.[40]

In addition to the persistence of VRE in livestock and healthy humans, a tiny, but growing, number of vancomycin-resistant *E. faecium* bacteremias (blood infections) had been occurring in hospitalized patients.[41] After the avoparcin ban, instead of decreasing as in the farm animals, VRE rates in hospitalized patients increased. In 2008 less than 1 percent of the *E. faecium* isolates were resistant, but one year later, resistance had increased to 1.6 percent. The resistance rates in 2012 and 2013 were 1.8 and 3.4 percent, respectively.*[42] The increasing use of vancomycin to treat ampicillin-resistant *E. faecium* infections in hospitals could explain the rising rates.[43] In 2013 an outbreak of vancomycin-resistant *E. faecium* with *vanA* resistance genes in Danish hospitals had health officials worried because of limited options to treat these infections.[44]

In Danish hospitals and primary care settings, vancomycin and other antibiotics were being increasingly used. From 1997 to 2013, the estimated total antibiotic use in hospitals (defined daily dose [DDD] / 100 occupied bed-days) increased more than twofold.*[45] In hospitals, cephalosporin use increased almost fourfold from 1997 to 2011 before decreasing the next two years.[46] In 2013 penicillin combinations were used 455 times as frequently as in 1997, and vancomycin use increased 6-fold in the same period.*[47] (However, these increases might be artifactual, since hospital lengths of stay decreased approximately 28%.)[48]

Antibiotic use in primary care increased 35 percent over the same 15-year period.[49] Penicillins and macrolides (e.g., erythromycin) were the most commonly used antibiotics in primary care settings.*[50] Despite increasing use of antibiotics in clinical medicine, Denmark consumed fewer antibiotics than other EU countries.[51] Antibiotic consumption in the entire European Union is discussed in Chapter 6.

In an effort to further reduce unnecessary antibiotic usage in clinical settings, the Danish Health and Medicines Authority issued guidelines in 2013 that narrowed the indications for their use.[52] One of the guidelines' aims was to ensure that critically important antibiotics were reserved for seriously ill individuals or used when no other alternatives were available. For example, primary care physicians were urged not to prescribe carbapenem antibiotics, because they are the antibiotics of last resort in the class of beta-lactam antibiotics (similar to penicillins and cephalosporins) to treat resistant *Enterobacteriaceae* such as *E. coli*.[53]

Carbapenem-resistant bacteria, which are believed to have originated in poultry, have been a worsening problem globally.[54] In many countries, young chicks are given third-generation cephalosporins to treat *E. coli* infections, leading to resistance. Cephalosporins have been used to treat infections, not for growth promotion, so the ban did not affect their use. Nevertheless, in Denmark, these drugs stopped being used in broiler production in the very early 2000s; in pig production, use ceased in 2010. But cattle production continued to use them to treat infections.[55]

The growth-promotion ban did not result in health problems in broiler chickens as it did in pigs. Poultry producers continued to use coccidiostats to prevent coccidiosis and necrotic enteritis.[56] Beginning in 1990, coccidiostat use fluctuated, with a spike around the time the ban was fully implemented.

The overall trend suggested decreasing use; however, no data was available after 2004.*[57]

Pig production changed dramatically in the 20 years spanning the ban. From 1993 to 2013, small producers (500 or fewer heads) decreased by 95 percent, and medium producers (501 to 4000 heads) decreased 76 percent. In contrast, in 1993 very large producers (10,000 or more heads) constituted only 2.5 percent of total pig suppliers, but in 2013, they constituted 46 percent of the pig producers.*[58]

Denmark's ban on growth-promoting antibiotics in the late 1990s did not adversely affect its pork production. From 1990 to 2007, annual pig-meat yield remained stable at approximately 0.078 million kg per 1000 heads. Two years after the 2006 EU growth-promoter ban went into effect, Denmark's yield increased 2 percent. But inexplicably, in 2008 yield decreased 6 percent, and in 2013 it fell almost 16 percent compared to 2007 levels.*[59]

The decreased yield did not adversely affect exports. From 1990 to 2013, fresh and frozen swine meat exports increased almost 60 percent. Imports, primarily from the Netherlands, Germany, France, Belgium, and other countries, decreased approximately 16 percent.*[60] Statistics Denmark had no explanation for outlier data.

According to the UN Food and Agriculture Organization (FAO), Denmark was the leading exporter of pig meat in 1996, but in 2000 it dropped to third place after the United States and the Netherlands. In 2011 it was tied for third place with the Netherlands.*[61] It is unclear whether Denmark's growth-promoter ban had an impact on its rankings in global pig-meat exports.

Denmark's avoparcin ban was highly successful in reducing rates of VRE in pigs and poultry. However, the ban had no apparent impact on reducing the rate of VRE in hospitalized patients with bloodstream infections. One explanation for this unexpected finding came from a genetic and statistical analysis suggesting that resistant *E. faecium* in hospitals is genetically distinct from the strains that asymptomatically inhabit the guts of animals and healthy humans in the community. Hospital-acquired VRE likely emerged from intense selective pressures in hospitals.[62]

Denmark provided intriguing findings, but to better understand the avoparcin ban's effect on VRE rates in pigs, poultry, and humans, an analysis of many countries was needed. Chapter 6 will examine the impact of the European Union's avoparcin ban and its subsequent ban of all growth promoting antibiotics.

CHAPTER SIX

The European Experience

The debate in Europe regarding a complete ban on growth-promoting antibiotics lasted for years. Acknowledging that pig and poultry farmers would be the hardest hit, Roger Cook, the director of the UK National Office for Animal Health, the organization representing manufacturers of animal medicines, said, "The ban will not apply to imports of meat from animals treated with these drugs outside the European Union, which will thereby gain a competitive advantage. We are in danger of crippling the industry and denying consumers home produce." Farmers pointed to Sweden, emphasizing that five years of higher rates of animal illnesses and mortality and an increase in therapeutic antibiotic use followed its ban.[1]

The public health community retaliated. The United Kingdom's Advisory Committee on the Microbiological Safety of Food, an independent group of microbiologists, issued a 700-page report concluding that antibiotics given to animals led to an emergence of some resistant bacteria that could infect humans.[2] However, the *extent* to which antibiotics given to animals contributed to antibiotic resistance in humans was uncertain. Additional surveillance and research were needed.[3]

In the late 1990s, scares involving unsafe animal feed undermined European consumer confidence. Amid falling meat prices, dwindling farmer income, and blockages on beef exports, the European Union announced plans to ban antibiotics in animal feed.[4] But the agriculture community was not convinced that livestock production was the main source of antimicrobial resistance.

Writing in *AgBioForum*, an agriculture-biotechnology journal, Ghislain Follet, the president of the European Federation of Animal Health Industries, discussed the findings of a 1999 European Commission report, drawn up by the Scientific Steering Committee of the European Union Directorate General XXIV, which outlined 14 key resistant organisms in human medicine.

The report recommended phasing out the use of all antibiotics as growth promoters.[5] Follet highlighted a subsequent, unrelated survey that asked 31 microbiology experts in the United Kingdom to rank each of the organisms in the 1999 EU Commission report in relative importance and likelihood of zoonotic origin. The experts concluded that 4 out of the 14 (*Campylobacter, Salmonella, Escherichia coli,* and vancomycin-resistant enterococci) were most likely to be of animal origin and that the contribution of these 4 organisms to the overall problem of antimicrobial resistance in humans should be very low.[6] Follet concluded that three times fewer antibiotics per kilogram weight were used in animals for feed purposes compared to therapeutic use in humans.[7] In addition, most antibiotics used for animals were older drugs, such as tetracyclines, different from the commonly used antibiotics for human use. His conclusion: "The European habit of banning antibiotic products is politically motivated rather than scientifically based."[8]

The EU policymakers, however, focused on a European Federation of Animal Health study, conducted by International Federation for Animal Health Europe, representing the European animal health industry, which found that in 1999 farm animals consumed 4,700 tons (35%) of all antibiotics administered in the European Union; of this total, 6 percent were given in feed as growth promoters. Humans consumed 8,500 tons (65%) of all antibiotics in the European Union.[9] Antibiotics as feed additives were politically unacceptable.

The European Ban

On March 25, 2002, the European Commission, the executive body of the European Parliament, introduced a proposal to ban the use of antibiotics as growth promoters. The decision was based on the precautionary principle.[10] David Byrne, the European Union's commissioner of health and consumer protection, spearheaded the effort.[11] Nine months later, the EU Commission for Health and Consumer Protection and the Agriculture Council reached an agreement on new rules to strengthen control of additives in animal feed, particularly antibiotics as growth promoters. "Anything to do with feed additives was politically toxic. This was a time when the European Union was dealing with mad cow disease and dioxin residues in meat and milk. The illegal additives were used to make producers richer," according to Byrne.[12]

In 2003 the European Parliament passed regulations prohibiting the use of antibiotics as growth promoters throughout EU member nations.[13] The new regulations set December 31, 2005, as the date when all antibiotics, except coccidiostats and histomonostats, would be prohibited as feed additives for growth-promotion purposes.[14] After January 1, 2006, veterinarians would be able to prescribe antibiotics only for sick animals.

Importantly, the Europeans did not address antibiotic use just in livestock but also in humans. The European Council, a body composed of the heads of state of the EU member nations, issued recommendations on November 15, 2001, on the prudent use of antimicrobial agents in clinical medicine. Its recommendations included gathering reliable, comparable data on the susceptibility of pathogens to antimicrobial agents; collecting data on prescriptions and use of antibiotics; educating health professionals on the appropriate use of antibiotics; and restricting the availability of systemic antibacterial agents to prescriptions only.[15]

Four years later, the European Commission issued its first report detailing the status of the European Council's recommendations.[16] At the national level, it found that almost all member countries had surveillance systems for antimicrobial use and antibiotic consumption in clinical medicine; however, lack of funding, unclear legal status, and privacy issues hindered full implementation. None of the countries were able to estimate the proportion of antibiotics sold without prescriptions, but at least seven countries allowed the practice. Most of the countries had guidelines on proper antibiotic use, but few monitored their impact. In addition, not all countries provided education on the appropriate use of antibiotics during health professionals' training.[17]

The commission's report influenced member nations and prompted them to act. In its second report, issued five years later, the commission found that 16 countries had developed national strategies to reduce antimicrobial resistance and an additional 8 were in the process of preparing them.[18] Only 4 member nations had no strategy in place or in process. Unfortunately, the problem of selling antibiotics without a prescription was reported in 16 countries.[19] Reasons for the continuation of this practice were not given.[20]

Antibiotic Use in Europe

At the multinational level, important surveillance systems in clinical medicine were being developed. For example, the European Committee on Antimicrobial Susceptibility Testing worked with the member nations to harmonize antimicrobial resistance monitoring by establishing breakpoints and standardized testing methods. The European Antimicrobial Resistance Surveillance Network (EARS-Net) collected resistance data from 800 laboratories in

28 countries. And the European Surveillance of Antimicrobial Consumption Network (ESAC-Net) implemented a European database to compare antibiotic use in clinical medicine across European nations.[21] As of 2011, the ESAC-Net included 27 European member states and two EEA (European Economic Area) non-EU countries (Iceland and Norway).[22]

ESAC-Net found that overall antibiotic use had significantly increased in community settings from 1997 to 2009; most antibiotic use occurred in community rather than hospital settings. Overall, penicillins were the most frequently prescribed antibiotics. Seasonal variations were observed: antibiotic use was higher in winter than in summer months.[23] Some countries, such as Denmark, Sweden, and the Netherlands, showed consistently low patterns of antibiotic use. Others, such as Greece, Cyprus, France, and Belgium, demonstrated continuous high-level use.*[24]

The types of antibiotics prescribed varied geographically as well. The Nordic countries judiciously used older narrow-spectrum penicillins and first-generation cephalosporins. In contrast, many southern European countries preferred the newer, broad-spectrum antibiotics. For example, in 2011 Greece, Cyprus, and Malta were the largest consumers of second-generation cephalosporins in Europe, and Italy and France consumed the most third-generation cephalosporins. There was a 190-fold difference in the use of cephalosporins between the Netherlands (0.04 defined daily dose per 1,000 inhabitants and per day—designated here simply as DDD) and Greece (7.58 DDD).*[25]

Vancomycin use in ambulatory and hospital settings varied from country to country as well, but not as much as cephalosporin use. Human vancomycin consumption data is not publicly available, and the European Centre for Disease Prevention and Control (ECDC) did not give permission to identify individual countries. Some countries were high users of the drugs; other countries were low users. There was an almost fourfold difference between the lowest vancomycin-using country (0.0146 DDD) and the highest-using country (0.0526 DDD).*[26]

ESAC-Net conducted a quality analysis of antibiotic use, employing drug-specific quality indicators. Quality was broadly defined as low consumption rates compared to high consumption rates. The analysis also found a north-south divide: the Nordic European countries and the United Kingdom showed higher-quality outpatient antibiotic use than did the southern European countries, such as Cyprus, Greece, Italy, Malta, and Spain. Belgium, France, and Luxembourg also demonstrated lower-quality antibiotic use. Eastern European countries were in between, showing moderate-quality use. Of note: the countries considered to have lower-quality antibiotic use also reported higher percentages of antibiotics sold without prescriptions.[27]

Reasons for the geographic differences were not given. But some countries' consumption patterns were based on national guidelines and did not, for example, use cephalosporins in community settings.[28] Also, cultural differences in patient expectations and physician practice patterns might explain some of the variations. Illness behavior is culturally shaped, influencing perceptions about feeling sick. Physician practice patterns could also be influenced by the culture and the medical system in which the physicians work.[29]

The Europeans established an antibiotic consumption surveillance system in veterinary medicine as well as in human medicine. In 2009, at the request of the European Commission, the European Medicines Agency launched the European Surveillance of Veterinary Antimicrobial Consumption (ESVAC).[30] Two years later, ESVAC published a report of antibiotic consumption in animals in nine countries from 2005 to 2009, the years before and after the growth-promoting ban.[31] Four of the nine countries, Czech Republic, Denmark, France, and the Netherlands, had the highest estimated weight of food animals to be sent for fattening or slaughter. Similar to Denmark, the Czech Republic increased its tetracycline use over the five years, but France and the Netherlands decreased theirs.[32]

In 2013, ESVAC released its report of sales data from 25 EU or EEA (European Economic Area) member nations. Tetracyclines (37%), penicillins (23%), and sulfonamides (11%) constituted the largest percentage of the 8,400 tons of antibiotics sold for primarily food-producing animals in 2011.[33]

In 2011 Germany, Spain, France, Denmark, Italy, the Netherlands, and Poland were among the largest pig producers in the European Union.*[34] But the magnitude of pig production did not necessarily correspond with antibiotic consumption. For example, in 2011 Italy produced almost half a percent fewer pigs than Denmark but consumed almost 20 times as much tetracyclines. Overall, Germany, Spain, and Italy were the largest consumers of antibiotics for livestock, using the highest amounts of penicillins and macrolides. But Poland surpassed Italy as one of the three top consumers of fluoroquinolones.*[35]

Third-generation cephalosporins were administered to eggs and day-old chicks to treat *E. coli* infections, but as with pig production, unexpected differences between countries were evident.[36] France produced 6 percent more poultry than Germany but consumed 1.5 times fewer third-generation cephalosporins. Poland and Spain were essentially tied in poultry production rates, but Spain consumed 4.5 times as much third-generation cephalosporins as Poland.*[37]

Antibiotic Resistance in Europe

The use of third-generation cephalosporin antibiotics in poultry has been blamed for the rise of resistant *E. coli* bloodstream infections in humans. Overdevest and colleagues in the Netherlands found that *E. coli* from chicken meat had a high prevalence rate (79.8%) of extended-spectrum β-lactamase (ESBL) resistance genes. Genetic analysis revealed a high degree of similarity between the ESBL resistance genes found in chicken meat and ESBL resistance genes found in *E. coli* from hospitalized patients with bloodstream infections.[38] The authors noted that the Netherlands is among the lowest users of antibiotics in clinical medicine but among the highest users in livestock, providing a good setting to examine the spread of antibiotic resistance from livestock to humans.[39]

Between January 2003 and December 2009, the number of *E. coli* bloodstream infections reported to EARS-Net by 281 laboratories in 28 European countries increased from 19,332 to 29,938, a 55 percent increase. During this time, *E. coli* resistance to third-generation cephalosporins increased from 2.7 to 8.2 percent. Extrapolating from this data, De Kraker and colleagues estimated that in 2007 alone, third-generation cephalosporin-resistant *E. coli* bloodstream infections were associated with 2,712 excess deaths and 120,065 extra hospital days. The trends suggested that these infections would likely increase rapidly in future years.[40]

EARS-Net has collected extensive antibiotic-resistance data in humans.[41] For example, the 2012 annual report showed 8 out of 30 countries with *E. coli* resistance rates against third-generation cephalosporins greater than or equal to 15 percent. These countries were Bulgaria, Cyprus, Greece, Hungary, Italy, Latvia, Romania, and Slovakia.*[42] Some of these countries, such as Greece, Cyprus, Romania, and Italy, were large consumers of second- and third-generation cephalosporins in humans.

From 2003 to 2012, *E. coli* cephalosporin resistance in Europe showed increasing trends. Resistance rates increased in Greece (almost threefold), Cyprus (threefold), Italy (more than fourfold), and Malta (sevenfold). Humans and livestock in Denmark and Sweden consumed little cephalosporins and had correspondingly low levels of resistance.[43] But inexplicably, some coun-

tries, such as France, had high levels of cephalosporin consumption and relatively low levels of resistance.* In humans, *E. coli* resistance to third-generation
cephalosporins was weakly correlated (R = 0.23) with cephalosporin sales
in livestock but strongly correlated (R = 0.63) with cephalosporin consumption in humans.*[44]

Unfortunately, European data collection from livestock is not as comprehensive as that for humans. Epidemiological surveillance monitoring of *Salmonella* and *Campylobacter* from livestock and food is mandatory, but it is
voluntary for *E. coli* and enterococcus.[45] As a result, only 11 countries reported
broiler chicken–derived *E. coli* resistance data against cefotaxime, a third-
generation cephalosporin. Belgium and Spain had the highest levels of resistance: 19.1 and 20.8 percent, respectively. Inexplicably, France and Germany,
the largest consumers of third-generation cephalosporins in poultry, had resistance rates about two and a half to three times lower than those of Belgium and Spain. Italy and the United Kingdom, the two other large consumers of third-generation cephalosporins in poultry, did not provide resistance
data for comparison. In general, *E. coli* resistance rates against cefotaxime were
higher in broilers than in pigs.*[46]

Data from six countries showed no correlation between cephalosporin
sales in livestock with *E. coli* resistance against cefotaxime in either broilers
(R = 0.116) or pigs (–0.186).*[47] However, *E. coli* cephalosporin resistance was
moderately correlated (R = 0.34) between broiler chickens and humans and
strongly negatively correlated (R = –0.66) between pigs and humans.* This data
does not establish causation; it merely suggests correlation at a broad population level.

The emergence of vancomycin-resistant enterococci (VRE) prompted the
European Union to ban avoparcin and other antibiotic feed additives in
1997.[48] In subsequent years, EARS-Net conducted extensive surveillance of
VRE in hospitals and laboratories in EU and EEA countries. Data over 10 years
(2003–13) on *Enterococcus faecium* vancomycin resistance rates in hospitalized patients showed considerable differences between countries and no ob-
vious trends. For example, Italy had an 83 percent decrease in VRE; Ireland
experienced a more than twofold increase.[49] Some countries, such as France,
the Netherlands, and Sweden, maintained consistently low levels of resistance.[50] The data showed no overall beneficial trends after the avoparcin
ban; VRE rates in Belgium, Cyprus, Denmark, Germany, Greece, and Ireland
fluctuated and increased in the years after the ban.* Human vancomycin

consumption and *E. faecium* resistance in 10 countries were strongly positively correlated (R=0.673).*

However, two studies in Germany and the Netherlands showed a decrease in VRE carriage in healthy people after the ban on avoparcin. The German study assessed fecal specimens from communities: 100 people in 1994, 100 people in 1996, and 400 people in 1997. (Germany banned avoparcin in 1996.) Of the 600 people tested, 21 carried VRE in their guts, but the percentage of VRE carriage dropped from 12 percent (12/100) in 1994, to 6 percent (6/100) in 1996, to only 3 percent (13/400) in 1997. In the Netherlands, fecal samples from communities taken in 1996 (117 humans) and 1999 (171 humans) demonstrated a 61 percent reduction in VRE carriage.[51]

The EARS-Net surveillance data on hospitalized patients showed that *E. faecium* had higher vancomycin resistance rates than *Enterococcus faecalis* had. In 2013, 9 countries out of 30 had *E. faecalis* resistance rates greater than 1 percent.[52] They were Bulgaria (3%), Czech Republic (4%), Greece (7%), Ireland (2%), Italy (1%), Latvia (7%), Luxembourg (7%), Portugal (3%), and Romania (1%).[53]

As with *E. coli,* less VRE data was collected from livestock than from humans. But one country stood out: Belgium. *E. faecium* from broilers in Belgium had a 9 percent resistance rate against vancomycin. The other countries either provided no data or had levels of resistance less than 2 percent.[54] There was not enough data to do a correlation assessment.

Pig and Poultry Production before and after the EU Ban

Did the ban have any effect on pig or poultry production in the European Union? The UN's Food and Agriculture Organization has provided annual global meat-production data by country and geographical region since 1961.[55] From 1996 to 2005, the United States and the European Union were the global regions producing the most pig meat.[56] During those years, the two regions differed by no more than 21 points. Beginning in 2006, when the EU antibiotic growth-promoter ban took effect, the US yield per carcass weight (animal) exceeded Europe's by an average of approximately 32 points.[57] Since 2006 the United States has consistently produced more pig meat per animal per year than the European Union.[58] Ratios of EU to US pig-meat yields, averaged 10 years before and 8 years after the ban, revealed an approximately 3 percent decrease in pig-meat production in Europe. This 3 percent decrease cost approximately 870 million euros per year in losses, or, in 2012 US dollars, approximately $1.1 billion per year.*

No relative changes were evident with chicken-meat production. However, it should be noted that coccidiostats and histomonostats in poultry were exempted from the ban. Since 1996 Europe has trailed consistently behind North America, South America, and Australia–New Zealand in chicken-meat production (yield per animal).[59] According to the UN Food and Agriculture Organization (FAO), the United States and Brazil have been the world's top chicken-meat exporters since 1996.*[60]

Health Care Costs of Antibiotic Resistance

In humans, considerable health care costs were associated with antibiotic-resistant infections. In 2009 an ECDC–European Medicines Agency Joint Working Group produced a report focusing on seven antibiotic-resistant bacteria that were frequently responsible for bloodstream infections in humans.[61] They determined that approximately 25,000 patients died from one of these infections in the European Union each year and that the extra health care costs and loss of productivity amounted to roughly 1.5 billion euros. For VRE and third-generation cephalosporin-resistant *E. coli* infections, an estimated 469,000 (18%) extra hospital days and 6,600 (26%) additional deaths occurred each year.[62] Extrapolating from the report's estimated yearly economic burden, the costs from VRE and third-generation cephalosporin-resistant *E. coli* infections alone were approximately 304 million euros, or, in 2007 US dollars, $411 million.[63]

Despite all their efforts, the Europeans concluded that their policies and actions were not enough to contain the rising threat of antimicrobial resistance. More rigorous measures were needed at the global level. In November 2011, the EU Commission launched a five-year action plan using a holistic One Health approach against antimicrobial resistance. The action plan proposed new efforts to ensure the appropriate use of antibiotics in both humans and animals, prevent infections from spreading, develop new antimicrobials, contain infection risks from international trade and travel, and promote innovative research.[64]

CHAPTER SEVEN

The Controversy in the United States

The Food and Drug Administration (FDA) obtained its authority to regulate drugs and foods after deadly scandals involving poisonous and tainted products. Public outrage led to change. The 1906 Food and Drugs Act forbade the marketing of drugs and foods that were adulterated or misbranded, but the FDA had no authority to *prevent* the practices that led to adulteration.[1] It could only punish the food producers after the fact. After 100 deaths from ethylene glycol, a poison added to an untested drug called Elixir Sulfanilamide in 1937, Congress passed the Federal Food, Drug, and Cosmetic Act of 1938, which required the FDA to monitor the safety of new drugs and forbid the sale of adulterated foods.[2]

However, the 1938 law did not give the FDA the authority to require *advance* proof that the chemicals used in food production were not poisonous. On July 6, 1945, Congress passed the Penicillin Amendment, requiring the FDA to ensure the safety and efficacy of penicillin-based drugs by certifying that batches of the drugs destined for market met the requirements for strength, quality, and purity.[3] But Congress also gave the FDA the authority to waive these requirements if doing so was considered safe; this waiver provided the FDA the flexibility to approve antibiotics for purposes other than treating infections, such as promoting growth in livestock. And indeed, the agency waived the requirements for batch certification for antibiotics intended as growth-promoting agents and as preventives against infection in livestock, in 1951 and 1953, respectively.[4] In essence, growth-promoting antibiotics in livestock production received a backdoor approval from the FDA before the problems of antimicrobial resistance became widely known.

From 1954 to 1968, Congress passed major food safety amendments. The Food Additives Amendment of 1958 required the FDA to approve new chemicals in foods, but the sole criterion for approval was *safety*—the chemicals could not be poisons. The FDA was not allowed to consider the potential benefits or risks of the chemicals.[5] There was one exception. Representative James Delaney of New York, the chairman of the committee overseeing the legislative reforms, inserted the famous Delaney Clause, stipulating that no additive could be considered safe if it was found to induce cancer when ingested by humans or animals.

In 1968 the Animal Drug Amendments were added and became the final piece of the food statutory framework, creating a single approval process for drugs and feed additives used in food animal production. Congress regarded animal drugs as food additives, meaning that only their safety could be considered for approval. The goal of the legislation was to ensure that the drugs were safe and effective in the animals and that any residues in the foods derived from the animals were safe for human consumption.

Any drug found to be carcinogenic would not be approved. Several companies had obtained FDA approval to market diethylstilbestrol (DES), a synthetic estrogen used as a growth-promoting agent in livestock and subsequently found to be carcinogenic in humans and animals, before the Delaney Clause was enacted. This situation presented the agency with a dilemma that took years to resolve.

Growth-promoting antibiotic use in livestock also presented challenges to the FDA, especially after Great Britain became the first country to implement partial bans, inspiring US public health activists to advocate for similar policies.[6] In 1966 the FDA formed the ad hoc Committee on the Veterinary Medical and Nonmedical Uses of Antibiotics to evaluate the various uses of antibiotics in livestock;[7] in 1970 it established a task force to address concerns about antibiotic resistance associated with their use. The task force recommended that the long-range goal should be to eliminate the use of subtherapeutic antibiotics that were also used to treat human diseases. Penicillin and tetracycline were the drugs of greatest concern.[8]

Congressional engagement with the issue of antimicrobial resistance grew slowly. In March 1971, the 92nd Congress held a hearing on the regulation of food additives and medicated animal feeds; much of the discussion centered on nitrates, nitrites, nitrosamines, and DES.[9] Antibiotic growth promoters were only briefly mentioned.[10]

Six years later, the Congressional Subcommittee on Agricultural Research and General Legislation of the 95th Congress held a hearing on the use of antibiotics in animal feed. Vermont Senator Patrick J. Leahy chaired the session. The hearing included statements from public health experts, consumer advocates, and agriculture and pharmaceutical industry representatives.[11] Dr. Donald Kennedy, commissioner of the FDA, said in his testimony that data showed conclusively that populations of people who worked around livestock receiving growth-promoting antibiotics had higher incidences of resistant organisms than people not exposed. "We are not arguing about a roadmap," said Kennedy. "We are arguing about traffic density. . . . The question is how often does it [the transfer of resistant microbes from animals to humans] happen?"[12]

Unable to attend the first day's hearing, Senator S. I. Hayakawa from California submitted a statement to the committee: "A fail-safe society is impossible, and before feed additives are withheld from use, economics should be considered for the good of the industry and the consumer." Senator Leahy replied, "We all agree that a fail-safe society is impossible. At the same time . . . the Government has certain responsibilities to remove dangers if possible while balancing the benefits and risks." Dr. Kennedy added, "We are dealing with the law in which Congress has already disposed of that problem . . . things like food additives, feed additives. . . . The public health considerations are more serious than the economic benefit considerations. And, in making that law, it told the Food and Drug Administration, `Please leave your hands off the question of risk-benefit balancing. Congress . . . has wisely chosen to keep those kinds of decisions in its own ball park and not to yield them up to regulatory agencies.'"[13]

The next day, Kansas senator Robert Dole commented on Dr. Kennedy's statement: "The revelation that was most shocking was in his [Dr. Kennedy's] answers to questions regarding [FDA] authority for taking action to ban these feed additives. . . . Once FDA approves a feed additive it should then be FDA's responsibility to prove what the new hazards are before taking action to ban the use of the approved additive. This proposed ban assumes a human health hazard that scientists cannot agree exists."[14] As the hearing continued, disagreements about the role of growth-promoting antibiotics in animal husbandry became intertwined with disagreements about FDA's statutory authority. Dr. Richard Novick, chief of the Department of Plasmid Biology, Public Health Research Institute, in New York, asserted that growth-promoting antibiotics were used to make up for the lack of good animal-husbandry practices: "The growth-promoting effect of antibiotics is seen only when animals are raised in suboptimal conditions—that is, in crowded, dirty, and heavily contaminated pens and feedlots. . . . When scrupulous care is taken . . . to raise animals, there is no growth promotion of antibiotics."[15]

But Dr. David A. Phillipson, president of the Animal Health Institute and vice president of Upjohn Company, disagreed: "Three factors are very important in animal husbandry practices; one is management, the second is genetics, and the third is disease control. . . . If you remove any one of those factors then the whole system is going to collapse. I dispute very strongly the assertion that animals are reared in unsanitary conditions. . . . Animal husbandry in the United States is the envy of the world . . . and it is not dirty and unsanitary. If it were, we wouldn't be able to produce at the level we are." Dr. Phillipson stated that there were no regulations or laws stipulating that products could be removed based on theoretical assumptions. He believed that the FDA was operating outside of the mandate of Congress: "I am absolutely certain that Congress, in its wisdom, never intended that we guarantee 100 percent safety. I don't think that's possible."[16]

But those sentiments did not reassure consumers. Mary Goodwin, chair of the Consumer Liaison Panel, Food and Nutrition Board, National Academy of Sciences, said, "As consumers we feel antibiotic feed additives should be proven safe before approval for human consumption. Why should we take unnecessary risks on human health when the consequences are unknown?" Dr. L. M. Skamser of American Cyanamid Company weighed in:

> FDA has said that when a hazard to human health exists, the law does not permit it to consider benefits. . . . In our opinion, this does represent a new interpretation of the law by FDA. . . . If the law does not permit consideration of benefit, then FDA must move promptly to prohibit the use of every agricultural chemical under their control, because some question of theoretical hazard can be raised about every single one of them. . . . No company can spend research dollars to develop new products which might be summarily banned because someone can theorize that a risk might exist.[17]

In a 1990 interview, Dr. C. D. VanHouweling, director of the Bureau of Veterinary Medicine, FDA, from 1967 to 1979, reminisced about the politics during that time: "Those hearings went on for years and years. I mean formal hearings, informal hearings, publications in the Federal Register. . . . We had studied this matter for years—and we said, `Why don't we just go ahead and do what the English did? Restrict the use to veterinarians' prescription?' So that's what we proposed to do. Dr. [Donald] Kennedy was happy with that. . . . But everybody else was opposed."[18]

The Congressional Office of Technology Assessment (OTA) published a report in June 1979 summarizing the evidence of the benefits and risks of low-level antibiotics in animal feeds and DES against the regulatory and public policy frameworks. The OTA report concluded that antibiotics in animal feed most likely had a disease-preventive effect, which was probably the primary reason for the increased weight gain of livestock. However, the growth benefit was offset by an increase in bacterial resistance to the drugs. The report stated that *Escherichia coli,* the bacteria common in the intestinal tracts of both animals and humans, posed the largest reservoir of drug resistance and could transfer its resistance genes to *Salmonella.* The report stated that the risk from resistant organisms of animal origin was not quantifiable, but the enormous pool of resistance genes in animals, and the ability of those genes to be transferred from one organism to another, threatened the therapeutic value of antibiotics against both human and animal diseases.[19] In assessing and quantifying the risks and benefits, the OTA report stated, "No common denominator is generally acceptable for comparing human illness and death with pounds of meat. Rather than using monetary values as a common denominator, opposing advocates usually seek to make their case or ridicule their opponents in the most exaggerated terms. For example, one advocate might say that if one life is saved, that is worth whatever it costs in decreased meat production, and Americans eat too much meat anyway."[20] The OTA report found that statutory authority limited FDA's decision making to be based strictly on scientific evidence of effectiveness and safety; the economic consequences of those decisions were not to be considered. In the case of growth-promoting antibiotics, the trade-off was between immediate economic benefits of livestock producers and meat consumers and future health risks. For DES, the report acknowledged that its recommendation focused on establishing a level of use and not on determining whether the substance should be banned. The report provided Congress with five options to consider:

1. Allow the FDA to decide the issue and ban the addition of low levels of penicillin and tetracycline in animal feed.

2. Enact legislation requiring the FDA to consider economic as well as scientific assessments of benefits and risks (the OTA admitted that it would be far more difficult to assess the monetary value of risks than the benefits).

3. For DES, enact legislation that eliminated the all-or-nothing approach to risk assessment and implement a target risk approach (e.g., by defining it as an added lifetime exposure risk of $1:10^6$ of developing cancer).

4. Require the FDA to decrease the therapeutic use of antibiotics in human and veterinary medicine as well as in food animal production (the OTA acknowledged that it would be easier to control antibiotics in animal feed than to regulate the practice of medicine and veterinary medicine).

5. Approve future drugs (i.e., antibiotics) only if they were at least as effective as those already approved.[21]

Congress was not convinced that the health hazards posed by the subtherapeutic antibiotic use in livestock were real and requested that more scientific data be collected.[22] The FDA was unable to ban the use of antibiotics as growth-promoting agents, but it was able to ban DES by invoking the Delaney Clause.[23] Over the decades, Congress, federal agencies, and scientific organizations have examined and reexamined the issue of growth-promoting antibiotics and antimicrobial resistance (appendixes A–C list many of these activities). In 1980 the National Research Council found that most of the studies on the subject were small and poorly controlled and that there was not enough evidence to prove or disprove that antibiotics in animal feeds were harmful to human health. It concluded that a comprehensive, all-encompassing study could not be done because of insurmountable technical difficulties.[24]

Frustrated by the lack of government action, Dr. Stuart B. Levy, a professor of molecular biology, microbiology, and medicine at the Tufts University School of Medicine, cofounded the Alliance for the Prudent Use of Antibiotics (APUA) in the early 1980s. Chapters sprang up worldwide. Its mission has been to improve antimicrobial use and to contain resistance, and it has been highly successful in generating media campaigns, raising professional and public awareness, and changing corporate policies.[25] Banning subtherapeutic antibiotic use in livestock has been one of its priorities.

For example, working in concert with animal-welfare groups and the Environmental Defense Fund, a nonprofit organization dedicated to preserving the environment, APUA helped persuade the McDonald's Corporation, the world's largest restaurant chain and a major purchaser of meat, to require its meat suppliers to stop using antibiotics as growth promoters.[26] Cargill and Tyson Foods, two of McDonald's largest meat suppliers, claimed that they would comply with McDonald's new standards, but the Animal Health Institute, an organization representing companies involved in veterinary health, stated that the decision was not based on sound science. A spokesperson for the American Meat Institute said, "This is not a decision motivated by science but by market research."[27]

National Antimicrobial Resistance Monitoring System

Of course, developing policies based on sound science requires good data. In the United States, the availability of good data on antibiotic use and resistance has been hampered by a combination of weak political will, limited funding, and proprietary interests. Despite all of its hearings and requested reports, Congress never appropriated funds specifically for antimicrobial resistance surveillance in animals or humans. Instead, senior administrators in federal agencies such as the FDA and the USDA acted on their own initiative to establish antimicrobial resistance surveillance programs.

For example, in May 1995 the FDA Veterinary Medical Advisory Committee (VMAC) met to discuss the use of fluoroquinolones in animal medicine. Most of the committee members agreed that fluoroquinolones were needed in food animals but should be available by prescription only. Several voiced concerns that fluoroquinolone use in food animals might lead to resistance in humans. The committee unanimously agreed that antimicrobial resistance levels should be monitored. Some members recommended monitoring antimicrobial resistance before and after the onset of fluoroquinolone use in food animals.[28]

Dr. David A. Kessler, pediatrician, lawyer, and FDA commissioner from 1990 to 1997, concurred with the VMAC recommendation and began the National Antimicrobial Resistance Monitoring System (NARMS) in 1996. NARMS is an interagency effort led by the FDA, the CDC, and the USDA. The program has three surveillance components: humans, food animals, and retail meats.[29] The FDA provides most of the funds, although the CDC and the USDA contribute resources as well. For fiscal year 2014, total funding for NARMS was $7.8

million ($4.516 million from the FDA, $2.009 million from the CDC, and $1.275 million from the USDA).[30]

In 1996 the CDC began collecting samples from humans from 14 sites, and in 2003 it expanded nationally. Public health laboratories would send human clinical specimens for further testing to CDC NARMS; these specimens were from individuals with gastrointestinal symptoms, presumably from foodborne illnesses.[31] The USDA's Agricultural Research Service (ARS) samples bacteria from food animals at slaughter plants, healthy animals on farms, and diagnostic specimens from sick animals.[32] The ARS began testing nontyphoidal *Salmonella* in 1997, *Campylobacter* in 1998, and *E. coli* and *Enterococcus* in 2000.[33] Since 2002 the FDA has been collecting samples from retail meats purchased at grocery stores in 11 states.[34]

NARMS data shows that nontyphoidal *Salmonella* has high rates of resistance against tetracyclines, particularly in isolates from retail meat such as chicken and pork chops. Isolates from humans revealed lower antibiotic resistance rates against nontyphoidal *Salmonella*. Tetracycline is not a drug of choice for *Salmonella* infections, and most *Salmonella* infections in humans resolve in five to seven days without antibiotics. For severe infections requiring antibiotics, the drugs of choice are typically fluoroquinolones, such as ciprofloxacin, or third-generation cephalosporins such as ceftriaxone.[35] The resistance rates against ciprofloxacin in chickens, swine, and their corresponding meats remained zero throughout all the testing years. In humans, however, it increased twofold. Resistance rates against ceftriaxone increased almost thirteen-fold and more than threefold, respectively, in chickens and chicken meat.* In humans, ceftriaxone resistance decreased almost twofold.[36]

For *Campylobacter jejuni*, NARMS collects data for chickens, chicken meat, and humans, but not for swine or pork chops. Data for chickens has been collected since 1997, but only since 2002 for chicken meat. As with *Salmonella*, resistance has been high against tetracyclines but has decreased approximately twofold during the years collected in chickens and chicken meat. Treatment against *Campylobacter* is not needed except when the infection is severe, and then especially in individuals with compromised immune systems. The drugs of choice are fluoroquinolones.[37] From 1998 to 2010, *Campylobacter* resistance to ciprofloxacin in isolates from chickens increased 2.5-fold. However, in chicken meat, resistance decreased to zero in 2011 after almost a decade of testing. In humans, *Campylobacter* resistance to ciprofloxacin increased in 2011 to 23.5 percent, a 1.1-fold increase from 2002.*[38]

There is no specific treatment for pathogenic *E. coli* gastrointestinal infections. In some cases, particularly O157:H7 infections in children, administering antibiotics is discouraged because it could lead to hemolytic-uremic syndrome, a deadly disorder caused by the lysis (i.e., rupture) of red blood cells, potentially leading to acute renal failure.[39] *E. coli* resistance against ceftriaxone tested 0 percent in 2002 and 2011 in humans.[40] Ceftriaxone resistance in chickens and chicken meat increased approximately 1.5-fold over the same period.[41] Tetracycline resistance decreased 1.5- and 1.1-fold in chickens and chicken meat, respectively; in humans, resistance increased almost 2-fold.*[42]

Since 2002 enterococcus resistance against vancomycin and linezolid has tested 0 percent in isolates from chickens, chicken meat, and pork chops. But resistance against quinupristin-dalfopristin has been high, particularly in chickens, increasing almost twofold from 2003 to 2006. Inexplicably, in chicken meat, quinupristin-dalfopristin resistance decreased almost twofold from 2002 to 2011.*[43]

Unfortunately, NARMS has not collected enterococcus resistance data from humans, in either communities or hospitals. In US communities, vancomycin-resistant enterococcus (VRE) has not been a problem. A study by McDonald and colleagues found a little *Enterococcus faecium* resistance to quinupristin-dalfopristin in 3 out of 334 outpatient human stool specimens submitted to state health department laboratories for routine cultures. The study did find a high prevalence of quinupristin-dalfopristin resistance in chicken meat, consistent with NARMS data. The authors concluded that despite 30 years of virginiamycin use in livestock, little enterococcal resistance to quinupristin-dalfopristin has developed in healthy humans.[44]

In US hospitals, however, VRE is a serious problem. Edelsberg and colleagues evaluated more than 80,000 hospital admissions of adults from 2007 to 2010 from 19 US hospitals. Of the 4,024 *E. faecium* clinical isolates tested, 87.1 percent were resistant to vancomycin. The CDC estimates that 77 percent of all US health-care-associated infections caused by *E. faecium* are resistant to vancomycin, contributing to approximately 10,000 infections and 650 deaths per year.[45]

Unlike Europe, the United States and Canada never licensed the use of avoparcin in food animals, because of concerns about its carcinogenic potential.[46] This fortuitous decision might explain why the epidemiology of VRE in the United States has been different from its epidemiology in Europe.[47]

Increased VRE prevalence rates in US hospitals preceded increased VRE prevalence rates in European hospitals by about a decade, even though the first VRE cases were reported in Europe.[48]

Hospital-associated *E. faecium* appears to have acquired high genome plasticity, meaning the microbe can undergo genetic changes with each generation. VRE has also acquired large numbers of resistance mechanisms and virulence factors, making treatment difficult.[49] One or two VRE clones caused the initial hospital outbreaks before evolving into multiple clones and becoming endemic in many US hospitals.[50]

In Europe, avoparcin was associated with resistant *E. faecium* in food animals; the microbes were primarily colonizers of human and animal intestinal tracts in community settings. But the hospital-associated group appears to be genetically distinct from the community-associated group. And 70 to 90 percent of the livestock isolates appear to be distinct but genetically related to the community-associated group.[51]

Surprisingly, genetic evidence indicates that hospital VRE clones may have come from other animals, just not the food animals everyone had assumed were the source. Instead, VRE may have evolved from dogs. *E. faecium* isolated from hospitalized patients appears to have a common evolutionary link with *E. faecium* isolated from dogs. One Danish study analyzed fecal swabs from 127 healthy dogs and found 20 *E. faecium* isolates resistant to ampicillin. One isolate had a sequence type belonging to VRE CC17. Only 14 of the dogs had been treated with antibiotics within six months of the study.[52]

A second study, conducted in Denmark and the United Kingdom, found ampicillin-resistant *E. faecium* (AREF) in 61 (29%) of 208 dogs analyzed. Only one out of 18 dog owners tested positive for AREF: a 10-year-old boy who lived with one of the dogs reportedly had close contact with it, with frequent petting and kissing, facilitating transmission of the microbe. Approximately one in every four of the dogs tested had AREF CC17, a potential precursor to VRE CC17, which has caused resistant hospital infections worldwide.[53]

USDA National Animal Health Monitoring System

Drs. James W. Glosser and Lonnie King, two senior administrators at the USDA, developed an animal disease surveillance system in 1990, separate from NARMS but also including antimicrobial resistance. A former veterinary epidemiologist with the CDC, Glosser was the USDA Animal and Plant Health Inspection

Service administrator from 1988 to 1991. King was the USDA deputy adminis-trator for Veterinary Services.[54] They initially called their program the National Animal Disease Detection System, but it was subsequently renamed the National Animal Health Monitoring System (NAHMS). They partnered with several universities to initiate training and begin pilot projects. King recalled their initial efforts: "NAHMS was a hard sell to agriculture, but eventually, we won out. NAHMS reports are now well accepted and have industry support. There was no congressional funding for the initiative. We wanted to make it noncontroversial, so it was a low-key but very strategic approach."[55]

Through NAHMS, the USDA collects antimicrobial resistance data in live-stock, including swine.[56] In 2006, 584 *Salmonella* isolates from swine tested negative for ciprofloxacin and ceftriaxone resistance.[57] Resistance to tetracy-cline was high. As of this writing, 2012 NAHMS *Salmonella* and *E. coli* data was not available.[58]

Campylobacter coli from swine showed significant resistance in 2006 to tet-racycline and erythromycin, but much lower, 3.3 percent, resistance to cipro-floxacin.[59] *C. coli* was not tested in 2012 because of budget cuts, and the mi-crobe was not considered a major foodborne pathogen, unlike *C jejuni*.[60] In 2006 swine *E. coli* isolates showed zero resistance to ciprofloxacin and ceftri-axone but very high (91.5%) resistance to tetracycline.[61]

From 2006 to 2012, no enterococcus isolates from swine were resistant to vancomycin or linezolid; testing against quinupristin-dalfopristin was not performed.[62] However, while NAHMS had not detected enterococcus resistance in swine, one study in Michigan isolated VRE from six pigs but not from other food animals or their human caretakers. It was the first time that VRE had been identified in food animals in the United States. Genetic analysis re-vealed that the VRE belonged to ST5 CC5, not CC17. Antibiotic use in owners was associated with VRE in pigs. One VRE-positive pig had received ceftiofur within 30 days of sampling; otherwise, there was no statistical association between antibiotic exposure in pigs and VRE presence.[63]

Unfortunately, neither NARMS nor NAHMS included full genome se-quencing of resistant microbes in their surveillance efforts. The technology is relatively new and expensive, since DNA sequencers only became widely available after 2006.[64] But without this critical information, fully under-standing the epidemiology of resistant microbes in animals, retail meat, and humans is extremely difficult.

CDC Report on Antimicrobial Resistance

The CDC used NARMS data and other sources in a 2014 report on antimicrobial resistance. The report estimated that more than 2 million people fall ill each year with antibiotic-resistant infections and of these cases, at least 23,000 die. The excess health care costs associated with these infections were estimated to range between $20 billion and $35 billion per year (2008 US dollars).[65]

The CDC report prioritized antibiotic-resistant bacteria into three categories: urgent, serious, and concerning. Nontyphoidal *Salmonella, Campylobacter,* extended spectrum β-lactamase producing *Enterobacteriaceae* (ESBL–*E. coli* and *Klebsiella*), and VRE were all listed as serious threats, but only nontyphoidal *Salmonella* and *Campylobacter* were categorized as threats from food animals.[66] Resistant *Enterobacteriaceae* and VRE were listed as health-care-associated infections. Resistant nontyphoidal *Salmonella* infections constituted approximately 8 percent of the total 1.2 million nontyphoidal *Salmonella* infections, and resistant *Campylobacter* infections made up approximately 24 percent of the total 1.3 million *Campylobacter* infections.[67]

The CDC did not provide estimates of health care costs for most of the resistant infections, but it did highlight total health care costs for nontyphoidal *Salmonella* infections. The estimated costs were approximately $365 million.[68] Eight percent of this would equal approximately $29.2 million. Robert L. Scharff, an assistant professor of consumer sciences at Ohio State University, calculated the economic burden from health care expenses resulting from foodborne illnesses in the United States.[69] Using an enhanced cost-of-illness model that included measures for lost quality of life, he estimated that the total mean cost in 2010 for nontyphoidal *Salmonella* and *Campylobacter* infections would be $11,391 million and $6,879 million, respectively. Applying the 8 percent and 24 percent estimates of foodborne infections resulting from resistant nontyphoidal *Salmonella* and *Campylobacter* would yield an estimated total cost of approximately $2.6 billion, or around 14 percent of the total health care costs, from these two microbes alone.

Antibiotic Use in the United States

Data on animal and human antibiotic use in the United States are less accessible than antimicrobial resistance data. For example, the FDA only began collecting data on antibiotic sales for food-producing animals in 2009 because Section 105 of the Animal Drug User Fee Amendments of 2008 required it to do so.[70] Unfortunately, this data is available only in aggregate; it is not separated by animal species. From 2009 to 2012, the most commonly used antibiotics in food-producing animals were tetracyclines and ionophores.[71] Total antibiotic use increased approximately 16 percent during that period.[72]

The USDA collects antibiotic-use data in food animals but primarily focuses on the method of administration (e.g., water, feed, injection) and the reason for use.[73] For example, in 1995 NAHMS data indicated that almost 93 percent of all grower and finisher pigs (final stage before slaughter) received antibiotics in their diets for disease-prevention purposes.[74] In 2006, 86.4 percent of grower and finisher pigs and 95 percent of nursery pigs (pigs weaned and placed in a nursery) received antibiotics in their feed for disease-prevention purposes.[75] Data on subtherapeutic antibiotic use for growth-promotion purposes was not included.

Apley and colleagues used swine-production data from the 2006 NAHMS swine study to estimate antibiotic use for growth promotion. Antibiotic-use data from 514 pig producers was extrapolated to represent approximately 24,398 production sites raising almost 57 million pigs. Using mathematical modeling, they estimated that approximately 256,235 kilograms of antibiotics were used in swine feed for growth promotion in one year in the United States.[76] Chlortetracycline (33%), bacitracin (28%), virginiamycin (10%), and tylosin (10%) were the most common antibiotics used for growth promotion. These antibiotics are related, respectively, to the following antibiotics used for humans: tetracycline, bacitracin (used in ointments), quinupristin-dalfopristin, and erythromycin. High rates of resistance against these antibiotics, particularly tetracycline, were evident in the NARMS and NAHMS data.

For humans, antibiotic-use data is proprietary and not available from federal agencies. However, the Center for Disease Dynamics, Economics, and Policy, a nonprofit policy institute in Washington, DC, and New Delhi, collects data for policy analysis and obtains antibiotic-use data under a license from IMS Health Xponent. The IMS Health data illustrates the variability of antibiotic use from state to state, a situation reminiscent of the variability between countries in Europe. For example, in 2010 Alaska had the lowest outpatient use of all classes of antibiotics, 0.510 dispensed prescriptions per person; Kentucky had the highest use, 1.196 dispensed prescriptions per person—a difference of 134 percent. In general, the Pacific and mountain states, particularly Alaska, California, and Hawaii, are low antibiotic-consumption states, while southern and central states such as Louisiana, Kentucky, Tennessee, and West Virginia are high antibiotic-consumption states. Differences in antibiotic use across the states were fairly consistent from 1999 to 2010 and were attributed to socioeconomic and cultural rather than medical factors.[77] The most frequently prescribed antibiotic in 2010 was azithromycin, a macrolide, commonly used for ear and respiratory tract infections.[78]

Americans use more antibiotics per capita than Europeans do.[79] From 1984 to 1996, Americans used 2 to 11 times more vancomycin per capita than was used in European countries such as France or the Netherlands, respectively.[80] High vancomycin usage would explain why VRE appeared about a decade earlier in US hospitals and why it has been such a serious problem in the United States.[81] Addressing antibiotic overuse in human medicine has been, in some ways, more difficult than in agriculture, although some academic medical centers have implemented "antibiotic stewardship" programs.[82] Some health experts estimate that 50 percent of outpatient antibiotic prescriptions may be unnecessary; in 2010 US health care providers prescribed 258 million courses of antibiotics. According to Dr. Levy, president of APUA, "Sometimes antibiotics have to be denied because they are not indicated—even if patients demand them. Getting physicians to change their prescribing behaviors will be hard, but fortunately, more professional medical groups are interested in this issue."[83]

US Poultry and Swine Production

The percentage of farms raising chickens has been steadily declining since the early twentieth century. From 1969 to 1992, farms with chickens decreased more than threefold. Most poultry are raised in the eastern half of the United States in large production facilities. In 2013 US broiler production totaled 8.52 billion head.[84]

The number of hog farms has also declined, from more than 300,000 operations in 1998 to less than 100,000 by 2012. Many small operations raise fewer than 100 pigs, but they constitute only 0.8 percent of the nation's inventory. At the other end of the spectrum, only 3.3 percent of the US hog operations raise almost 62 percent of the total inventory. These operations have more than 5,000 animals each.[85]

Despite the reduction in the number of farms, the yield in pounds of pig meat and particularly broiler meat produced per year has increased over the past 50 years. From 1963 to 2013, pig-meat production increased approximately 50 percent.[86] For broilers, the increase in production was more than 600 percent.[87]

In spring 2013 porcine epidemic diarrhea virus, a deadly disease causing severe vomiting and diarrhea, began killing millions of pigs and sent pork prices to record highs.[88] The virus slipped through US borders and spread over a dozen states. By early 2015, however, the epidemic was brought under control through new vaccines and herd immunity. US pork prices dropped as herds recovered.[89]

Increases in meat production have allowed the United States not only to meet its population's food demands but also to help other nations meet their food needs through the international market. In 1995 US pork exports surpassed imports.[90] From 1995 to 2012, pork exports increased more than 580 percent. Imports increased only 24 percent.[91] After Brazil, the United States is the second-largest exporter of poultry meat. From 1990 to 2013, US poultry-meat exports increased 544 percent.[92] There were zero poultry-meat imports until 1991, after which a small trickle began.[93] In 2013 approximately 122 million pounds of poultry meat were imported, compared to 7,364 million pounds exported.[94]

Americans enjoy relatively inexpensive meat. Adjusting for inflation, retail prices for broiler meat and pork have slowly decreased with time. Poultry has been consistently less expensive than pork; from 1980 to 2013, the retail price-per-consumer price index for poultry decreased approximately 16 percent. Over the same period, pork decreased approximately 6 percent.[95] Chicken meat is lower in fat and cheaper than pork. Not surprisingly, consumption of chicken meat in the United States has increased while pork consumption has been comparatively flat or has decreased. From 1980 to 2012, chicken-meat consumption increased almost 77 percent, and pork consumption decreased 20 percent.[96]

Americans pay less for meat, at least for pork chops, than some Europeans do. According to LABORSTA, the International Labor Office database on labor statistics, operated by the UN International Labour Organization, the retail price of a pork chop in the United States from 1990 to 2008 was generally lower than prices in the United Kingdom, Sweden, and Denmark. The exception was the United Kingdom in 1991: the price there was $7.05 per 1 kilogram pork chop compared to $7.42 in the United States. Otherwise, over the 18 years, pork chop prices increased 38 percent in the United Kingdom, 10 percent in Sweden, and 4 percent in Denmark. In the United States, the price decreased 1 percent.[97]

US Congress, FDA, and a Presidential Executive Order

Prestigious medical journals such as the *New England Journal of Medicine* have published editorials calling for an end to the use of nontherapeutic antibiotics in livestock.[98] Medical and public health professionals have lobbied policymakers for years. So far, efforts in Congress to ban subtherapeutic antibiotic use in livestock have been unsuccessful.

In 2007 congresswoman Louise Slaughter, a microbiologist and public health professional representing the 25th district of New York, introduced the Preservation of Antibiotics for Medical Treatment Act. It died in committee. She reintroduced the legislation in subsequent sessions of Congress, and the bill was unsuccessful each time.[99] However, medical and public health advocates won the battle for public opinion. The American media have published many articles emphasizing the health hazards of subtherapeutic antibiotic use in livestock, and editorials have demanded action. The politically explosive term "factory farm" is one example of the negative public opinion of large-scale food animal production.[100]

In 2011 the Natural Resources Defense Council, the Center for Science in the Public Interest, the Food Animal Concerns Trust, Public Citizen, and the Union of Concerned Scientists filed a lawsuit to require the FDA to prove that the use of subtherapeutic antibiotics in livestock was safe.[101] Two district courts ruled in their favor, prompting the FDA to propose a voluntary initiative banning growth-promoting antibiotic use in livestock.[102] The voluntary initiative would keep antibiotics available for treating, preventing, or controlling illness in livestock, but only under the supervision of veterinarians.[103] According to Dr. Richard Carnevale, vice president of regulatory, scientific, and international affairs for the Animal Health Institute in Washington, DC, "The FDA needs the cooperation of pharmaceutical companies and agriculture if it wants to implement changes in livestock antibiotic use. If they tried to push through a mandatory regulation, they would have to go through a long and deliberative administrative process to scientifically document a risk to human health for each type of antibiotic. The companies could respond saying that they don't agree. The process could take years. Voluntary guidelines were the most prudent way to go. All 26 of the involved pharmaceutical companies have stated that they would cooperate."[104]

The American Veterinary Medical Association supported the new rule but expressed concerns that small and remote farmers would have a hard time abiding by it, since fewer than 10,000 large-animal veterinarians are practicing in the United States. The Center for Science in the Public Interest was unhappy with the voluntary guidelines, stating that they were "tragically flawed." On July 24, 2014, in a two-to-one decision, the US Second Circuit Court of Appeals in New York overturned the 2012 rulings, stating that the FDA was not required to hold hearings regarding the safety of subtherapeutic antibiotics in livestock. A *New York Times* editorial severely criticized the court decision, calling it "appalling," and rallied readers to demand that supermarkets and restaurants stock only meat and poultry raised without antibiotics.[105]

On September 18, 2014, President Barack Obama issued Executive Order 13676, "Combating Antibiotic Resistant Bacteria," the first executive order to address antibiotic resistance. It established a national strategy with goals that included the improvement of antibiotic resistance surveillance, using a One Health approach; the elimination of using medically important antibiotics for livestock growth promotion; and the strengthening of educational programs and antibiotic stewardship programs in hospitals, clinics, and long-term-care settings.[106]

Concomitantly, the President's Council of Advisors on Science and Technology (PCAST) issued a report on combating antibiotic resistance. PCAST found that the United States spent $450 million per year on antibiotic resistance. The funding has been split between various departments, including Health and Human Services, Agriculture, Defense, and Veterans Affairs, and 75 percent of the funds have gone to basic and applied research. Human and animal antibiotic-resistance surveillance programs have been severely underfunded and lack the necessary advanced genomic technologies that would enable epidemiologists to fully understand the emergence and spread of microbial resistance. PCAST recommended, among other things, that federal spending double to $900 million per year with an additional $800 million per year to incentivize pharmaceutical companies to produce new antibiotics.[107]

In response to PCAST's recommendations, President Obama included a historic investment to address antibiotic resistance in his 2016 budget proposal. He proposed spending $1.2 billion across four departments: the Department of Health and Human Services ($1 billion), the Department of Agriculture ($77 million), the Department of Defense ($85 million), and the Department of Veterans Affairs ($75 million).[108] The increase in funds would improve surveillance, reporting capabilities, risk assessment, research innovation, and other initiatives. It was up to the 114th Congress, with a Republican majority, to approve the proposed increase in spending.[109]

CHAPTER EIGHT

International Challenges

In 2001 the World Health Organization (WHO) published *Global Strategy for Containment of Antimicrobial Resistance* after convening a series of expert workshops and consensus meetings in the late 1990s and 2000 on antimicrobial resistance.[1] The report cited the World Health Assembly Resolution of May 1998, which urged member nations to address the worsening crisis.[2] Unfortunately, the launch of WHO's global strategy in Washington, DC, coincided with the September 11 terrorist attacks, which overwhelmed news coverage of the event.[3]

WHO's global strategy included reducing disease burden and spread, improving antimicrobial use in humans and food-producing animals, strengthening health systems and disease surveillance, and promoting drug and vaccine development.[4] The report prompted some countries to develop national plans, but the overall response was weak. Many low- to middle-income countries were reluctant to develop or enforce laws banning over-the-counter sales of antibiotics because many people had no access to health care providers.[5]

The tepid global response had repercussions. In 2008 the emergence of a new multi-drug-resistant bacterium from India generated worldwide concern. A 59-year-old Indian man with chronic medical problems, who had lived in Sweden for many years, traveled to the Punjab region in India, where he became ill, required surgery, was transferred to several hospitals, and received multiple courses of intravenous antibiotics. From this patient, a resistant *Klebsiella pneumonia* possessing new resistance genes was identified. One of them was NDM-1.[6]

The New Delhi metallo-β-lactamase 1 (NDM-1) gene conferred resistance to virtually all antibiotics. The NDM-1 gene was on a plasmid allowing it to be transferred from microbe to microbe. A subsequent epidemiological study identified the gene in *K. pneumonia* and *Escherichia coli* isolates from people in India, Pakistan, and the United Kingdom. Most of the people in the United

Kingdom with microbes possessing NDM-1 had traveled to India or Pakistan in the previous year.[7] In other words, NDM-1 was spreading.

In April 2014 WHO published a second report on the global situation of antimicrobial resistance.[8] This report received more attention than the 2001 report.[9] It used data from national and international surveillance networks of antimicrobial resistance and from the scientific literature since 2008. A total of 114 countries out of 194 WHO member states (59%) provided data for at least one bacterial species. Seven resistant bacteria, excluding *Mycobacterium tuberculosis,* were selected as being of greatest international concern.[10]

Of these seven microbes, only *E. coli* and nontyphoidal *Salmonella* were listed as zoonotic (i.e., food animal) in origin. The report stated that the magnitude of transmission from animal reservoirs to humans remained unknown and probably varied depending on the bacterial species. It listed 11 countries that collected surveillance data on *Salmonella, Campylobacter, E. coli,* and *Enterococcus* from humans, animals, and food. Only Denmark collected data from healthy humans.[11]

WHO established a Global Foodborne Infections Network (GFN) in 2001 to promote UN member states' capabilities to collect surveillance data on foodborne diseases and to reduce antimicrobial resistance in foodborne pathogens.[12] Unfortunately, the GFN has been hindered by a lack of international standards and policies in sampling, testing, and reporting—resulting in an inability to harmonize different countries' surveillance systems. WHO subsequently initiated an advisory group to help integrate the surveillance of antimicrobial resistance across countries and established a tripartite agreement with the Food and Agriculture Organization (FAO) and the World Organization for Animal Health to address antimicrobial resistance in humans and animals.[13]

Despite all the limitations, the 2014 WHO report listed antibiotic resistance rates in the member countries that provided data. Some countries stood out: India and Pakistan reported *E. coli* third-generation cephalosporin resistance rates of 85 percent or higher. These two countries also reported *E. coli* fluoroquinolone resistance rates of 85 percent or higher, as did Bangladesh, Kenya, and the Solomon Islands.[14] Peru reported the highest nontyphoidal *Salmonella* fluoroquinolone resistance rate in the world, 96 percent; but many countries, including India and Pakistan, did not provide data for this microbe.[15]

In 2010 India, China, and the United States were the world's largest, second-largest, and third-largest consumers of antibiotics in humans, respectively, according to an analysis of national pharmaceutical sales data. International trends in human use have been rising; from 2000 to 2010, global antibiotic consumption increased 36 percent. Cephalosporin and fluoroquinolone consumption increased dramatically over the decade, particularly in Germany, China, and India.[16]

Purchasing and consuming antibiotics without a prescription (i.e., self-medication) in many countries have contributed to resistance. Factors reinforcing the practice of self-medication include lack of access to medical care, weak or nonexistent laws limiting antibiotic availability to prescription only, and illegal sales.[17] A literature review of more than 100 articles and community surveys spanning almost 40 years (1970–2009) found that nonprescription antibiotic use in countries outside North America and northern Europe was widespread, ranging from 19 to 100 percent. Nigeria and Sudan had the highest rates of nonprescription antibiotic use: 100 percent each. Bangladesh and Vietnam had the second- and third-highest rates of 86 and 62 percent, respectively.[18]

Even for individuals who seek medical care, appropriate antibiotic use is not guaranteed. In many countries, health care providers prescribe antibiotics inappropriately because of high patient demand for antibiotics and fear of missing something serious.[19] Improving physician prescribing practices has been a tremendous challenge, especially in the care of children, who are high users of the medications. Many physicians do not weigh health implications for the general population in their decisions to prescribe antibiotics.[20]

Chile

Unfortunately, countries that try to improve antibiotic use do not necessarily succeed. In 1999 Chile banned over-the-counter sales of antibiotics and required physician prescriptions. Antibiotic use decreased over two years, from 2000 to 2002, but lack of enforcement led to a return to preban levels.[21] Chile's efforts to curtail antibiotic use did not extend to its aquaculture industry. Salmon fish farming is one of Chile's largest industries and employs, directly and indirectly, more than 50,000 people. In 2008 Chile used almost 350 times more antibiotics than Norway, the largest salmon producer in the world.[22] Chile's aquaculture industry has been struggling with infectious salmon anemia, a viral disease responsible for killing millions of fish, and has been relying extensively on three antibiotics, oxytetracycline, oxolinic acid, and florfenicol, to limit the spread of bacterial infections. Environmentalists complain that unsanitary fish farms cause the illnesses.[23] Industry representatives insist that they have been working with Chilean government officials to solve the problems.[24]

Bangladesh and Kenya

In Bangladesh, more than 55 percent of prescribed antibiotics are cephalosporins. The most frequent conditions that receive antibiotics are acute respiratory tract infections, watery diarrhea, trauma, and gastrointestinal distress. Ciprofloxacin, a fluoroquinolone, is used extensively for treatment of suspected gonorrhea, resulting in substantial resistance. More than one-quarter of purchased antibiotics are for children suffering from pneumonia or diarrhea; about 230,000 children in Bangladesh die from diarrhea annually. As in other developing countries, antibiotics are available without a prescription, and self-medication is common since physician visits are expensive.[25]

In Kenya, antibiotics are available without a prescription and are frequently misused. As in much of Africa, there is a shortage of microbiology facilities and diagnostic capability, and people are afraid of serious outcomes without antibiotics. Self-medication is frequent since access to health care is limited. In livestock, antibiotics are not typically used for growth promotion but are used for therapeutic applications. Most antibiotics used in livestock are tetracyclines, and multi-drug-resistance predominates on small farms—almost double the rate on large farms. Kenya has limited veterinary services. As with humans, most antibiotics for animals are purchased over the counter from retail pharmacies.[26]

Pakistan

In Pakistan, studies in hospital and community settings suggest that physician antibiotic prescriptions are frequently inappropriate. One study examined trends of antibiotic use in pediatric patients in a hospital in Karachi. Of the 161 patients studied from November 2010 to May 2011, most were admitted with acute gastroenteritis (i.e., fever, nausea, and vomiting) and were prescribed third-generation cephalosporins as empiric therapy. The authors could not find any justification for this practice. The inappropriate therapy continued at discharge even though stool and blood cultures tested negative.[27]

In Pakistan's community settings, the situation is even worse. Physicians readily prescribe antibiotics whether or not they are indicated. Many Karachi residents do not bother seeking medical care and self-medicate for symptoms of pharyngitis (sore throat) and gastroenteritis because antibiotics are readily available without a prescription. And as soon as they feel better, people stop taking their antibiotics, further promoting resistance. The most commonly used antibiotics are penicillin and macrolides.[28]

There is no surveillance program for antibiotic use in livestock in Pakistan.[29] Chickens and buffaloes are the most commonly consumed food animals. A Pakistani study testing fecal specimens found more resistance in *E. coli* isolates from poultry than from buffaloes. Both groups of animals harbored resistance genes in their feces, but only the poultry were exposed to antibiotics in their feed. The buffaloes consumed antibiotic-free grass and natural fodder, but their fecal specimens exhibited resistance. The study authors attributed these findings to buffaloes' ingesting water contaminated with antibiotic residues.[30]

Pakistan's fish farms are at an early stage of development and have no recorded history of antibiotic use. Mixtures of fresh poultry and cattle manure are typically applied to newly constructed ponds and applied multiple times during the year to boost zooplankton and phytoplankton production. Wastewater contaminated with fecal materials commonly flows into the fish farms. The survey of aquaculture ponds in Pakistan found a variety of antibiotic-resistant genes with bacteria resistant to tetracycline, trimethoprim, penicillin, erythromycin, and other antibiotics. The researchers concluded that manure and wastewater contributed to the high levels of antibiotic resistance found in Pakistan's aquaculture.[31]

Peru

Peru's extremely high rate of nontyphoidal *Salmonella* fluoroquinolone resistance is difficult to explain with the limited data available. In 2007 Venezuela, Argentina, and Chile, but not Peru, were the largest users of quinolone antibiotics. However, from 1997 to 2007, Peru experienced the largest increase in total antibiotic usage of eight South American countries studied.[32] Approximately 25 percent of antibiotics are available without a prescription in Peru, but most caregivers seek professional medical advice for children's illnesses. Unfortunately, physicians frequently prescribe antibiotics inappropriately for mild, self-limited illnesses.[33]

In Peru, data for livestock is minimal. Peru is not a major livestock producer, and small, rural Peruvian farms are not major users of antibiotics. Most of the antibiotics used on dairy farms were oxytetracyclines, penicillins, and trimethoprim-sulfamethoxazole drugs, not fluoroquinolones.[34]

India and China

Although many countries report high antibiotic use and resistance, India and China deserve special attention. They have the world's largest populations, more than 1 billion people each, and they consume the most antibiotics. In 2014 the *New York Times* singled out India for creating the perfect conditions for untreatable bacteria to emerge: abysmal sanitation and widespread antibiotic misuse.[35]

On July 15, 2014, a front-page *New York Times* article highlighted that open defecation in India was causing severe malnutrition and stunting in children. Sixty-seven percent of rural Indian households, involving hundreds of millions of people, defecate outdoors. Many Indians in rural areas defecate in the open despite economic growth and government construction of latrines. The people prefer defecating outside and find the practice to be more pleasurable and desirable than using latrines. The problem has not been an issue of poverty; the rural poor in Bangladesh, Southeast Asia, and Sub-Saharan African countries use latrines.[36] Instead, the problem has been cultural preference.

Five months later, a second front-page *New York Times* article described outbreaks of "superbugs" in India that were killing tens of thousands of newborns. Bacteria resistant to virtually all antibiotics have been spreading in India's sewage, soil, water, animals, and people. Rather than improve sanitation and hygiene to prevent infections, Indians rely on antibiotics to fight them.[37]

Between 2005 and 2009, antibiotics sold for human use increased approximately 40 percent. During this time, sales of cephalosporins rose 60 percent, increasing more than the other antibiotics. Antibiotic consumption in India typically peaks during the postmonsoon season between July and September, suggesting a link with the incidence of dengue fever.[38] But a virus causes dengue fever, so antibiotics prescribed for this illness are inappropriate.

As with Pakistanis, when Indians seek medical care, antibiotics are typically prescribed inappropriately. Some physicians prescribe antibiotics to all patients presenting with fevers, and many patients expect antibiotics to be prescribed whenever they feel ill. Making matters worse, pharmacists have an incentive to sell as many antibiotics as possible because they generate profits.[39]

In late 2014 the Indian Medical Association announced the launch of a national awareness program on the overuse of antibiotics. The organization planned to hold lectures to educate the public and train physicians to educate peers on the proper use of antibiotics. The Indian government, however, had no plans to take action against widespread human misuse of the drugs.[40]

But the government did target livestock. In 2012 the Indian Health Ministry inserted a rule in the 1945 Drug and Cosmetics Act that required a time period during which livestock must be kept off antibiotics before entering the human food chain. Poultry and mammals would have to be kept off antibiotics for 28 days before slaughter. Aside from this rule, essentially no regulations of antibiotic use in food animals exist in India, and there is no data on antibiotic use in livestock.[41] But compared to other countries, India consumes relatively little meat. From 1990 to 1992, Indian meat consumption, including bovine and poultry meat, was less than 20 kcal/cap/day, whereas China's meat consumption was more than 200 kcal/cap/day. India's low meat consumption has been largely attributed to religious preferences. More than 80 percent of Indians practice Hinduism, which promotes vegetarianism; 13 percent are Muslim, and 2.3 and 1.9 percent are Christian and Sikh, respectively. Approximately 40 percent of Indians do not eat meat, constituting the largest fraction of vegetarians in the world. Thirty-one percent do not consume animal proteins of any kind, but 9 percent of the vegetarians do consume eggs.[42] Muslims do not eat pork.

India is the world's largest producer and consumer of milk, producing more than 130 million tons in 2012–13, a 128 percent increase from a decade earlier. Most of the milk comes from buffaloes, not cows. From 1992 to 2012, the Indian buffalo population increased almost 30 percent. During the same decade, the cattle and pig populations decreased 7 and 20 percent, respectively. Goats and sheep increased 17 and 28 percent, respectively, but India's poultry population increased approximately 137 percent.[43]

Unlike India, China regulates nontherapeutic (e.g., growth-promoting) antibiotic use in food animals, a practice widely implemented since the mid-1970s. In 1989 China's Ministry of Agriculture issued regulations stating that only antibiotics not used in human medicine could be used as feed additives, and antibiotics could not be given during specified time periods before slaughter. But despite the regulations, more than 6,000 to 8,000 tons of unapproved tetracyclines have been given each year to at least 36 million cattle, 500 million pigs, and 70 billion poultry.[44]

By 1999 China used at least four times as much antibiotics in livestock as the United States. In 2007 China produced approximately 210,000 tons of antibiotics, and almost half of it went into livestock feed. The animals excrete vast amounts of antibiotic residues in their feces. Chinese swine generate an estimated 618 billion kilograms of manure each year.[45] Large-scale swine farms (10,000 animals per year) extensively use nontherapeutic and therapeutic antibiotics; manure samples from these farms have been found to produce antibiotic-resistant gene concentrations up to 28,000 times higher than manure samples from antibiotic-free farms. Not surprisingly, high levels of antibiotic residues and resistant microbes have been found in animal wastewater, surface water, and manure around farms and feedlots in various Chinese provinces.[46]

China never approved avoparcin for use in its livestock, and vancomycin-resistant enterococci (VRE) have not been detected in the country's farms, food animals, or meats—with two exceptions. First, in 2001, Japan identified two resistant *Enterococcus faecalis* strains from chicken meat imported from China. Second, from 2008 to 2013, almost 1,900 food animals in Hong Kong were swabbed for the presence of VRE.[47] One batch from pigs collected in January 2013 tested positive for vancomycin-resistant *Enterococcus faecium*, which was of the genetic lineage ST6/CC5 and possessed vanA, erm(B), and tet(M) resistant genes. The ST6/CC5 lineage was different from the VRE lineages isolated from hospitalized Chinese patients; however, it was very similar to the VRE lineages isolated from swine in Denmark, Portugal, Switzerland, Spain, and the United States and from healthy humans in Denmark.[48] How this particular lineage of VRE appeared in Hong Kong was unknown.

Besides terrestrial agriculture, China has a long history of aquaculture dating back more than 2,000 years; large-scale production began in earnest after the People's Republic of China was founded in the mid-twentieth century. In 1979 total aquaculture production was 1.23 million tons; by 2003 production was more than 30 million tons, an almost twenty-five-fold increase. Carp farming constitutes about 75 percent of the species produced, followed by bream, tilapia, crab, eel, and others. Pond cultures, primarily around the Yangtze and Pearl river basins, account for almost 71 percent of the fish-farming systems.[49] Chinese aquaculture uses penicillin, streptomycin, erythromycin, and other antibiotics in fish or egg disinfection and bath treatments. Antibiotic use in aquaculture has been associated with contamination of river and surface water. Downstream runoff from these sources is the likely reason antibiotics are found in coastal waters.[50]

The Chinese also use large amounts of antibiotics in humans. China consumes about 10 times as much antibiotics per person as the United States does. As in India, antibiotics are often inappropriately prescribed for viral infections. Approximately 75 percent of patients with influenza are given antibiotics, as are 80 percent of hospitalized patients.[51] A systematic review of antibiotic use in China found that more than 50 percent of outpatients received antibiotics. Level-one (i.e., community) hospitals in less developed western Chinese provinces used significantly more (57.4%) antibiotics than higher-level hospitals (47.3%) in more developed eastern provinces.[52] Another study analyzing antibiotic prescriptions in outpatient and inpatient settings found similar findings: prescription rates were lowest in Beijing and highest in Jilin, an underdeveloped inland province. More than 70 percent of the antibiotics prescribed were cephalosporins, penicillins, fluoroquinolones, and nitroimidazoles. Glycopeptides (i.e., vancomycin) and linezolid were not used.[53] Nearly 4,000 outpatient antibiotic prescriptions were analyzed, and almost 61 percent of them were considered inappropriate, according to the standards of the "Principles of Clinical Use of Antibiotics" issued in 2004 by the Chinese Ministry of Health in an effort to promote judicious use.[54] Seventy-five percent of more than 2,000 inpatient antibiotic prescriptions were also considered inappropriate.[55]

Financial incentives appear to be major drivers for high antibiotic prescription rates in China. Beginning in the 1980s, the Chinese government decreased financial support to hospitals to only 8 percent, forcing them to generate most of their income by charging patients for health care services and drugs. More than 50 percent of hospital revenues come from drug sales, of which 47 percent are antibiotic sales; hospitals typically mark up prices an additional 15 percent.[56] Most physicians work as salaried employees in hospital clinics and receive bonuses, constituting a sizable part of their salaries, for meeting drug-sales targets. Pharmaceutical company kickbacks further increase physician incentives to write antibiotic prescriptions. One study found that physicians prescribed significantly fewer antibiotic prescriptions for cold and flu symptoms and virtually no expensive antibiotics when auditors, posing as patients, stated that they would buy their medications "elsewhere."[57]

The Chinese public regards antibiotics as a panacea for all their ills and frequently demands them even when they are not indicated. They perceive newer antibiotics to be more effective and prefer to have them administered intravenously or by injection. Until 2004, antibiotics were available over the counter, and some families kept a supply at home. Antibiotics are also available illegally on the streets.[58]

China established several surveillance systems in an effort to understand the extent of antibiotic resistance. In 1994 the Peking Union Medical College Hospital began surveying intensive care units in 15 hospitals across the country. Four years later, Fudan University started the Shanghai Antibacterial Surveillance Network, which collected routine clinical microbial data annually from more than 10 hospitals. The Shanghai network expanded to include 20 hospitals; in 2005 it became known as CHINET. In addition, the Chinese Ministry of Health established the MOH National Antibacterial Resistance Investigation Network (MOHNARIN), the country's largest surveillance network, involving 80 member hospitals across China.[59] These surveillance systems found that antibiotic resistance in China was high and rapidly rising. Resistance rates of some bacteria, such as extended-spectrum β-lactamase-producing *E. coli* and quinolone-resistant *E. coli,* were 60 percent.[60]

One study analyzed more than 100 VRE specimens from 12 hospitals in China. Ninety-five percent of the isolates were *E. faecium.* Almost all the VRE isolates' DNA included clonal complex 17 (i.e., CC17), suggesting a common ancestor for the VRE infections in Chinese hospitals. VRE CC17 is a hospital-adapted subpopulation that has been responsible for the majority of hospital outbreaks of VRE infections worldwide.[61]

China initiated health care reforms in 2009 with the goal of ensuring basic health care for all Chinese by 2020.[62] These reforms included policies promoting the rational use of antibiotics. Physicians' pay was separated from drug sales in 2010, but for hospitals, funding sources aside from drug sales were not offered. In August 2012 the Chinese Ministry of Health implemented strict regulations for the medical use of antibiotics.[63] The measures included education programs for medical students and practitioners, task forces, audit and inspection systems, and targets for antimicrobial management. All hospital presidents were expected to chair antibiotic task forces, restrict hospital formularies, and credential health care providers for the right to prescribe specific antibiotics. Severe penalties would be implemented if the goals to limit antibiotic use were not met.[64]

During the first two years of implementation, excellent hospitals were lauded and failures were publicly criticized. Economic sanctions were imposed on some physicians, and poorly performing hospital presidents were dismissed. The policies had an impact: from 2011 to 2012, antibiotic sales decreased from 25 to 17 percent. For hospitalized patients, antibiotic prescriptions decreased from 68 to 58 percent, and outpatient antibiotic prescriptions decreased from 25 to 15 percent.[65] No other country has implemented regulations as draconian as China's to reduce antibiotic use in its health care system.

CHAPTER NINE

Environmental and Pharmaceutical Discoveries and Challenges

Advances in science and technology are shedding new light on antibiotic resistance, suggesting that the issue is far more complex than the simple overuse or misuse of antibiotics. Microbiological techniques developed in the late nineteenth and early twentieth centuries were useful for identifying disease-causing pathogens but limited in understanding microbial ecosystems. Some estimate that only 1 percent of all soil microbes have been identified, because most do not grow in laboratories.[1]

Environmental Discoveries

Metagenomics is a new field in which DNA is extracted directly from environmental specimens (e.g., soil, water, manure), completely bypassing the need to culture and identify bacteria. The genetic material can be analyzed using a variety of techniques, such as polymerase chain reaction–based methods or deep sequencing technologies. A downside to metagenomics, however, is that the original microbes from which the extracted DNA came are not necessarily known. In addition, contamination in DNA extraction kits and other laboratory reagents can lead to misleading results.[2]

Nevertheless, the technique has revealed intriguing findings. For example, low doses of antibiotics in the environment seem to have *hormetic* (i.e., beneficial) effects as signaling agents for bacteria. Scientists had assumed that bacteria use antibiotics as chemical weapons against competitors. But low doses appear to induce bacteria to change behavior, such as increasing movement, producing biofilms, or synthesizing chemicals, suggesting that antibiotics might serve as regulators or signaling agents in microbial ecosystems.[3]

Many microbes live in environments without anthropogenic (i.e., human-induced) antibiotic exposures yet still have antibiotic resistance genes. These resistance genes are everywhere: in soils, in secluded caves, in deep oceans, in Antarctic lakes, and in arctic snows, as well as in human and animal guts. Researchers used metagenomics to compare DNA extracted from environmental, human, and animal specimens collected from sites around the world with antibiotic resistance genes from the Antibiotic Resistance Genes Database.[4] They found that DNA from chicken guts, cow guts, and arctic snow had the lowest number of DNA matches with antibiotic resistance genes compared to those from soils and human feces.[5]

Antibiotic resistance genes appear to be ancient and to predate the selective pressures of modern antibiotic use. Scientists analyzed DNA sequences from Alaskan permafrost sediments dating back to the Late Pleistocene. Permafrost is defined as ground that remains at or below zero degrees Celsius for at least two years. They found highly diverse groups of genes encoding resistance to tetracycline, penicillin, and vancomycin, among other antibiotics. Questions remain, however, about whether the microbes in permafrost are dormant or metabolically active, potentially influencing when they evolved and acquired their resistance genes.[6]

To assess whether levels of antibiotic resistance genes in soil have changed over time, researchers in the Netherlands conducted metagenomic studies of archived soil samples dating from 1942 to 2008. These samples came from rural sites across the country. Information about chemical use, manure applications, or water irrigation use was not available, but the archived soil samples had no apparent contamination or DNA degradation. The researchers found increasing concentrations of antibiotic resistance genes with time, especially those conferring resistance to tetracyclines. Antibiotic resistance genes were especially high for specimens from pig manure, compared to cattle or sheep manure, correlating with the high use of antibiotics in pigs. They expressed surprise at the finding, given the European Union's ban on antibiotic growth-promoting agents, but noted that tetracycline use increased during the years after the ban.[7] This finding is consistent with the postban experiences in the United Kingdom and Denmark. Therapeutic antibiotic use increased after the implementation of the 2006 EU growth-promoter ban.

Microbes share genetic material through horizontal gene transfer (i.e., microbial sex), and this process appears to occur readily between bacteria in soil and those in manure.[8] Manure's role in the spread of antibiotic resistance genes is only beginning to be understood. The application of manure to soil as fertilizer for crops is widespread in many countries.[9] In the United States, large concentrated animal feeding operations (CAFOs) produce massive amounts of manure.[10] In a report investigating the environmental impact of CAFOs, the US General Accounting Office (GAO) estimated that a large hog farm, with as many as 800,000 hogs, generated more than 1.6 million tons of manure annually, which is more than one and a half times the waste produced by about 1.5 million residents of Philadelphia, Pennsylvania, each year.[11] From 1982 to 2002, large hog farms and large broiler chicken farms in the United States increased in number of farms by 508 percent and 1,187 percent, respectively, and produced thousands of tons of manure annually.[12] Researchers believe that CAFOs alter microbial ecosystems and promote the transfer of resistance genes through direct application of manure to soil, airborne drift of contaminated dust, animal waste runoff into water systems, animal waste in slaughterhouses, and animal waste on food.[13]

Sewage treatment plants might also contribute to the spread of antibiotic resistance genes. A metagenomic analysis of influent and effluent from the largest secondary sewage treatment plant in Hong Kong in 2011 and 2012 revealed high resistance-gene diversity and concentrations in influent wastewater. Both municipal and hospital wastewater contributed to influent wastewater. Sewage treatment effectively removed 99.82 percent of the resistance genes in the effluent wastewater; however, many persisted in the removed sludge.[14] Wastewater sludge containing antibiotics is sometimes used as fertilizer on agricultural soils or released to rivers.[15] In Germany, 30 percent of sewage sludge containing significant concentrations of nonmetabolized antibiotics from hospitals and households is used in agriculture.[16]

Terrestrial antibiotic use is not the only selective pressure source for increasing antimicrobial resistance. Antibiotics are also heavily used in aquaculture. The depletion of the ocean fisheries has facilitated a dramatic increase in aquaculture in both developed and developing countries. Norway originated salmon aquaculture in the 1970s, and since then, fish farming has spread worldwide. Fish farms are typically large anchored pens or cages that release substantial amounts of wastes into coastal waters.[17] In 2012 approximately 42.2 percent of the 158 million tons of fish consumed originated in commercial fish farms.[18]

Unlike low-dose antibiotic use in livestock to promote growth, antibiotics are used in aquaculture primarily to prevent disease, as the enclosed, unhygienic, and densely populated environments in which fish are raised are highly stressful and result in reduced immune system function. In developing countries, contaminated seawater frequently mixes with industrial, human, and animal wastewaters, turning the coastal environments into veritable cesspools. Strong epidemiological and molecular evidence suggests that fish pathogens, such as *Aeromonas,* share antibiotic resistance genes with human pathogens such as *Escherichia coli* and pass from aquatic to terrestrial environments. One study tested catfish, shrimp, salmon, tilapia, trout, and swai purchased in US stores but originating in fish farms from 11 countries. The researchers found 47 antibiotic residues even though some of the fish were marketed as "antibiotic-free." Some countries are implementing strict regulations on antibiotic use in aquaculture and enforce maximum residue levels for their products.[19]

The immense reservoir of resistance genes in aquatic and terrestrial environments, collectively known as the "resistome," forms a global network. Many common human pathogens, such as *Salmonella typhimurium* and *E. coli,* appear to have recently acquired antibiotic resistance genes that are identical to those found in the soil. Scientists speculate that intense selective pressure from extensive antibiotic use in clinical medicine and animal agriculture likely promotes resistance gene exchange between human pathogens and other microbes in the global resistome.[20]

Some newly acquired antibiotic resistance genes appear to come with a fitness cost: a reduced ability to reproduce. Depending on the environment, bacteria that acquire antibiotic resistance genes exhibit a reduced growth rate. There are exceptions, of course, and some resistant genes confer no disadvantages. Others confer a slight advantage in fitness.[21]

The general assumption by individuals advocating for a reduction in antibiotic use is that decreased use would lead to a reduction in antibiotic resistance. The rationale is that susceptible bacteria outcompete resistant bacteria. But some studies in community settings suggest that decreasing antibiotic use alone does not necessarily lead to a reduction in resistance. For example, one study showed that an 85 percent reduction in the use of trimethoprim-containing drugs over a 24-month period in Kronoberg County, Sweden, resulted in no apparent change in *E. coli* or other bacterial resistance rates. The authors speculated that there might be a minimal fitness cost associated with trimethoprim resistance. In a second study, a national program to reduce sulfonamide resistance in *E. coli* in the United Kingdom led to a 98 percent reduction in sulfonamide prescriptions (320,000 prescriptions per year in 1991, 7,000 prescriptions per year in 1999). Despite the dramatic decrease, *E. coli* resistance remained high, possibly because of a genetic linkage between the sulfonamide resistance gene and other resistance genes. In a third study, researchers found clarithromycin-resistant enterococcus even though one to three years had passed since the use of antibiotics to eradicate *Helicobacter pylori* infections.[22]

In contrast to the negative studies, Finland experienced a reduction in resistance in response to decreased antibiotic use. In late 1991 Finland implemented a national policy to reduce the use of macrolide antibiotics for skin and respiratory infections in outpatient settings after an increase of erythromycin-resistant *Streptococcus pyogenes* raised alarms. The *Finnish Medical Journal* and lectures at national and local meetings were used to educate general practitioners about the new policy. From 1991 to 1992, macrolide antibiotic use decreased approximately 43 percent and remained low for the duration of the five-year study. Two years after the policy change, *S. pyogenes* resistance rates began to fall. At the end of the study, resistance had decreased almost twofold, from 16.5 percent to 8.6 percent.[23]

In a hospital-based study, the Hunter Holmes McGuire Veteran Affairs Medical Center, affiliated with the Medical College of Virginia in Richmond, began a hospital-wide restriction of clindamycin use in March 1994 in response to an outbreak of clindamycin-resistant *Clostridium difficile* infections in hospitalized patients. In the months after the new policy was implemented, clindamycin use decreased 87 percent. Twenty months later, only 39 percent of the *C. difficile* isolates were resistant to clindamycin, in contrast to 91 percent resistance before the new policy was implemented.[24]

In 1996 the New York Hospital Medical Center of Queens implemented a hospital-wide policy to restrict the use of virtually all cephalosporins. The results were mixed. Cephalosporin use decreased 80 percent, but imipenem use, especially in intensive care units, increased 140 percent. The hospital experienced a 44 percent reduction in nosocomial ceftazidime-resistant *Klebsiella* infections. Concomitantly, it had a 68.7 percent increase in imipenem-resistant *Pseudomonas aeruginosa* infections.[25]

In livestock, Denmark's 1995 ban of the glycopeptide growth promoter avoparcin led to reductions of resistant enterococci. Cecal specimens from broiler chickens showed a highly significant reduction in glycopeptide-resistant *Enterococcus faecium*. In this study, however, isolates from pigs were essentially unchanged, in contrast to the findings presented in chapter 5. In the Netherlands, the 1997 EU ban of avoparcin in livestock led to a statistically significant decline over the subsequent two years in vancomycin-resistant enterococci in broiler chickens, pigs, and healthy humans.[26] Germany also experienced declines of VRE after its avoparcin ban in January 1996.[27] These studies, discussed in greater detail in chapter 6, illustrate the complexity of bacterial ecology and antimicrobial resistance. Some show a benefit in restricting antibiotic use, while others do not.

Further complicating the issue is the finding that wildlife harbor microbes possessing antibiotic resistance genes. Waterfowl, birds of prey, foxes, rabbits, feral pigeons, wild boars, rodents, and other animals have been found to carry resistant microbes, such as *E. coli,* in their guts.[28] The microbes possess genes conferring resistance against tetracycline, penicillins, cephalosporins, aminoglycosides, sulfonamides, and other antibiotics.[29]

How antibiotic resistance genes developed in wildlife assumed to have never been exposed to antibiotics is unclear, but some researchers speculate that these animals likely came into contact with water or soil contaminated by municipal wastewater sludge or livestock manure used in agriculture. Supporting this hypothesis is the fact that *E. coli*–producing extended-spectrum β-lactamases have been found to share identical gene sequences in wildlife, domestic animals, and humans. For example, a resistant *E. coli* clone, specified as B2-O25b:H4-ST131 with a CTX-M-15-type β-lactamase enzyme, is spreading worldwide and has been found in humans, companion animals,[30] and a Glaucous-winged gull caught at the Commander Islands off the remote far eastern Russian Kamchatka peninsula.[31]

Bird droppings are ubiquitous in urban and rural settings, and bird migration could serve as an important vector in spreading antibiotic-resistant genes around the globe. If wild animals, especially migrating birds, serve as reservoirs for antibiotic resistance genes, then efforts to reduce resistance could be much more difficult. Studying antibiotic resistance in the environment should include not only the external environment but also internal environments. The microbiome is the massive assemblage of competing and cooperating microbes that coevolved on and within hosts' bodies. These microbes thrive in mouths, ear canals, gastrointestinal tracts, nasal passages, skin, and female vaginas. Microbiomes keep hosts healthy by playing a critical role in immunity.[32]

In 2007 the National Institutes of Health launched the Human Microbiome Project after the human genome sequencing project yielded surprising results about human bodies: it is estimated that they contain ten times as many microbial cells as human cells. In essence, humans and other animals are "supraorganisms" composed primarily of microbes. This realization has dramatically changed perceptions about health and disease. For example, Dr. Martin Blaser, the director of the Human Microbiome Program at New York University, believes that the overuse of antibiotics in humans (especially children) and animals has caused parts of their microbiomes to disappear, contributing to the development of not only antibiotic resistance but also many chronic conditions such as allergies, diabetes, obesity, certain cancers, and asthma.[33]

However, a nationwide population-based cohort study in Sweden found no link between fetal and early childhood antibiotic exposure and subsequent development of asthma. More than 180,000 children with asthma who had received antibiotics in utero or in early childhood were compared with siblings who did not have asthma. The increased risks disappeared when siblings were included in the analyses, suggesting that risks associated with antibiotic use are due to confounding factors shared within families.[34]

Livestock microbiomes have also been studied. Danzeisen and colleagues examined the effects of monesin (an anticoccidial drug used in poultry production), virginiamycin, and tylosin for 35 days on cecal microbiomes and metagenomes of broiler chickens. They found that monesin given alone led to reductions in gut microbes such as *Enterococcus, Lactobacillus,* and *Roseburia,* a microbe negatively correlated with mouse obesity. The reduction in *Roseburia* might explain some of the weight gain seen in poultry treated with monesin. Treatments combining monesin with tylosin or virginiamycin led to reductions in *Enterococcus* but increases in *E. coli.* Metagenomic analyses revealed no significant differences in antibiotic resistance gene counts between control and treatment groups.[35]

An examination of swine intestinal microbiomes revealed dramatic differences related to gut location. Piglets were divided into control groups and treatment groups receiving low doses of chlortetracycline, sulfamethazine, and penicillin in their feed until euthanasia. The ileum (i.e., the section of the small intestine closest to the colon) had reduced microbial diversity compared to the rest of the gut. Antibiotic treatment altered the microbiome by increasing some bacteria, such as *E. coli,* while decreasing others, such as *Helicobacter* species. Fecal analyses alone did not reveal the microbial changes in the guts in response to antibiotics, demonstrating the importance of sampling microbes in vivo to fully understand how growth-promoting antibiotics work. Metagenomic analyses showed diverse and abundant antibiotic resistance genes in both medicated and nonmedicated pigs.[36]

Looft and colleagues studied the effects of low-dose antibiotics on the intestinal microbiomes of piglets. They divided a litter of six piglets into two groups: three raised with an antibiotic feed additive containing chlortetracycline, sulfamethazine, and penicillin commonly given to swine and three raised without the additive. They collected fecal samples intermittently during the 21 days of continuous treatment. They found a striking difference in the percentages of *Proteobacteria* (specifically *E. coli*) populations between the two groups: 1 percent in the untreated versus 11 percent in the treated animals. The subtherapeutic antibiotic treatment increased the abundance and diversity of resistance genes above the baseline levels of resistance genes that the untreated swine microbiomes already harbored.[37] Subtherapeutic antibiotics also appeared to decrease *Bacteroidetes* populations, increase *Ruminococcus* species, and increase energy production genes, all of which are associated with improved feed efficiency and growth.[38] At the same time, subtherapeutic antibiotics promoted virulence genes and gene-transfer capabilities.[39] Understanding how antibiotics alter microbiomes is critical for improving global human and animal health.

Pharmaceutical Challenges

Given the enormity of the global resistome and the tons of antibiotics used in medicine and agriculture each year, the emergence of antibiotic resistance should not be a surprise.[40] Soil bacteria, particularly the Actinomycete class, have either directly or indirectly provided the vast majority of the antibiotics used by societies. The soil bacteria already possessed antibiotic resistance genes; selective pressures from widespread antibiotic use over decades facilitated their expression and spread. Nevertheless, antibiotic resistance might not have become such a severe public health crisis if new effective antibiotics had been continually replacing the old, ineffective ones. Instead, the pipeline dwindled dramatically over three decades because the natural products, the "low-hanging fruit," starting with penicillin, had already been harvested. Adding to the problem, significant economic and regulatory disincentives discouraged pharmaceutical companies from investing hundreds of millions of dollars into research and development.[41] Many companies curtailed or abandoned their efforts altogether. Others might have relied too much on the unfulfilled promise of genomics. Since the early 1980s, there has been an eightfold decrease in the number of new antibiotics approved in the United States.[42]

Coinciding with pharmaceutical disengagement, changes in federal grant funding for basic biomedical research likely made matters worse. The problem was not necessarily a lack of funding; from fiscal year 1998 to FY 2003, Congress almost doubled the National Institutes of Health budget to $27.1 billion. NIH funding peaked in FY 2010 at almost $31 billion before declining slightly in subsequent years.[43] The problem was that the NIH became more conservative in deciding who received grant funding.

Beginning around 1990, demands for federal biomedical research grant funding dramatically increased because of a rapid expansion in the scientific workforce. Graduate students and postdoctoral fellows conduct most of the basic biomedical research in the United States and are paid by principal investigators' research grants. Principal investigators are usually established scientists who stick with their successful formulas rather than to explore risky new areas of research. The trainees devote their most productive years bouncing from fellowship to fellowship in hypercompetitive environments that suppress original thinking, creativity, risk taking, and cooperation. Risky projects can generate new insights needed for the development of novel drugs, but unfortunately most of them fail.[44]

In 2014 only 3 percent of NIH biomedical grant recipients were 36 years of age or younger; in contrast, in 1980 that number was 16 percent. Slowdowns in employment opportunities in academia, government, and pharmaceutical and biotechnology industries discourage young scientists. As a result, many opt out of biomedical research careers entirely despite years of investment in education and training.[45] Ultimately, the public loses.

On March 1, 2013, a federal sequestration began that required the NIH to cut $1.55 billion (5%) of its FY 2013 budget. All programs, projects, and activities sustained cuts, affecting every area of medical research and further decreasing grant funding availability. These cuts resulted in the funding of even fewer new research ideas.[46]

The reluctance of pharmaceutical companies to support risky ventures that may or may not result in new products might explain why virtually all newly approved antibiotics have been variants of preexisting drugs. Up until about 30 years ago, governments were generally more willing to make long-term investments in efforts with high failure rates, such as basic biomedical research.[47]

Europe has made efforts to boost antibiotic development. In 2008 the European Union and the European Federation of Pharmaceutical Industries and

Associations (EFPIA) partnered in the Innovative Medicines Initiative (IMI); each donated 1 billion euros ($1.23 billion) to stimulate new drug development. From this total, approximately 224 million euros ($275 million) was dedicated to a new antimicrobials initiative. Five EFPIA companies are taking part in the IMI antimicrobial resistance program: AstraZeneca, Basilea, Glaxo-SmithKline, Johnson & Johnson, and Sanofi.[48]

In the United States, the Infectious Diseases Society of America (IDSA) has taken a lead role in pushing for new antimicrobial drugs by proposing legislative and funding solutions. In 2010 it launched its "10×'20 Initiative" calling for the development and approval of 10 new, effective, and safe antibiotics by 2020. On September 19, 2014, Dr. Barbara E. Murray, president of the IDSA, testified before the Health Subcommittee of the US House of Representatives Energy and Commerce Committee, stating that the rise of antibiotic-resistant bacteria coupled with the market failure to develop new antibiotics constituted a public health emergency. She expressed her appreciation to Health Subcommittee members Congressmen Phil Gingrey and Gene Green for their leadership in helping enact the Generating Antibiotic Incentives Now (GAIN) Act, which had been included in the larger Food and Drug Administration Safety and Innovation Act of 2012.[49]

The aim of the GAIN Act was to provide economic incentives for pharmaceutical companies by ensuring an accelerated FDA approval process and market exclusivity for new antibiotics. In her written statement, Murray outlined additional legislative and federal agency efforts to spur new antimicrobial therapeutics and diagnostics. Unfortunately, as of 2013, only four large multinational pharmaceutical companies remained in antimicrobial research and development. Small pharmaceutical and biotechnology companies and a few larger ones in Japan conduct the work.[50]

In September 2014 the President's Council of Advisors on Science and Technology (PCAST) released its report on combating antibiotic resistance. It found that federal spending addressing the issue was limited. As of FY 2014, approximately $450 million (or $1.40 per American) was allocated across four federal agencies (Health and Human Services, Veterans' Administration, Defense, and Agriculture); approximately 75 percent is allocated for basic and applied research, and the rest is used for antibiotic resistance surveillance and antibiotic stewardship programs. The NIH allocates approximately $250 million in funding for research directly focused on antimicrobial resistance. PCAST recommended that total research funding be increased by $150 mil-

Legislative Efforts to Promote New Antimicrobials

- Generating Antibiotic Incentives Now (GAIN) Act of 2012. Added five years of exclusivity for new antibiotics that treat serious or life-threatening infections.

- Antibiotic Development to Advance Patient Treatment (ADAPT) Act of 2013, H.R. 3742. Would address regulatory hurdles by creating a new FDA approval pathway allowing companies to use smaller clinical trials to test new antimicrobial drugs. Approval would be for the population most in need of therapy.

- Developing an Innovative Strategy for Antimicrobial Resistant Microorganisms (DISARM) Act of 2015, H.R. 512. An earlier version of HR 512 was HR 4187, the DISARM Act of 2014. Would provide Medicare add-on payments for antibiotics used in hospitals to treat life-threatening infections.

- Protecting Access to Medicare Act (PAMA) of 2014, H.R. 4302. Extended Medicare payments to physicians and improved diagnostic test reimbursement. Signed by president on April 1, 2014.

Source: B. E. Murray, "21st Century Cures: Examining Ways to Combat Antibiotic Resistance and Foster New Drug Development," written statement to the Energy and Commerce Committee, Health Subcommittee, U.S. House of Representatives, September 19, 2014.

lion to a total of $400 million per year over seven years, culminating in a rigorous evaluation.[51]

PCAST also found, after discussions with government and industry experts, that the expected economic impact from the GAIN Act would be limited and would provide little to no incentive for pharmaceutical companies to invest in new antibiotic development. It recommended that the Biomedical Advanced Research and Development Authority,[52] which had already invested approximately $2.5 billion in research and development for medical countermeasures, expand its antibiotic development program beyond material threat agents and include urgent public health priorities. It estimated that a federal investment of $800 million annually in a newly established Antibiotic Incentive Fund would be needed to yield approximately one new antibiotic per year. PCAST also recommended that newly approved antibiotics receive higher federal reimbursement rates in outpatient and inpatient settings to increase economic incentives for pharmaceutical companies.[53]

One pharmaceutical industry expert agreed with one of PCAST's recommendations. Dr. Barry Eisenstein, senior vice president of Scientific Affairs,

Federal Agency Efforts to Promote New Antimicrobials

- National Institute for Allergy and Infectious Diseases (NIAID). Established Antibacterial Resistance Leadership Group (ARLG), which focuses on antibacterial drug and diagnostic test development.

- Centers for Disease Control and Prevention (CDC). Proposed Detect and Protect against Antibiotic Resistance Initiative, a bacterial isolate library to be used by researchers for developing new antibiotics and diagnostics.

- Defense Threat Reduction Agency (DTRA) and Defense Advanced Research Projects Agency (DARPA). Provide funding for antibiotic research.

- Biomedical Advanced Research and Development Authority (BARDA). Established Broad Spectrum Antimicrobials (BSA) program and since 2010 awarded more than $550 million to companies for antibiotic development.

Source: B. E. Murray, "21st Century Cures: Examining Ways to Combat Antibiotic Resistance and Foster New Drug Development," written statement to the Energy and Commerce Committee, Health Subcommittee, U.S. House of Representatives, September 19, 2014.

Cubist Pharmaceuticals, stated, "We need to fix the root causes of this innovation drought. In the hospital, government payments are bundled into a pre-established Diagnostic Related Group (DRG) where there is no individual reimbursement for life-saving antibiotics. A carve-out from Medicare's DRG inpatient payment system or new reimbursement mechanism for the hospital setting may be the single most impactful thing that can be done to jump-start the development of new antibiotics."[54]

But even if new antibiotics were developed, resistance would inevitably follow. Since human bodies are primarily microbial cells, future antimicrobial therapy would have to protect the human microbiome by targeting pathogens and sparing important commensal (i.e., coexisting and beneficial) microbes.[55] Traditional antibiotic therapy typically kills both pathogen and commensal microbes, periodically resulting in secondary infections such as *C. difficile* colitis or vulvovaginal candidiasis.

Some biologists advocate for a new therapeutic armamentarium beyond antibiotics. For example, virtually all bacteria produce bacteriocins, biologically active peptides with highly specific bacteria-killing properties, which are different from antibiotics. These potent peptides are already used as food preservatives and preventives in food-animal production; they are nontoxic and could be developed for therapeutic use in humans.[56]

Another therapeutic option is bacteriophages (a.k.a. phages), which are viruses that infect specific bacteria and kill them. Discovered in the early twentieth century by Frederick Twort, a British bacteriologist, and Felix d'Herelle, a French microbiologist, bacteriophages have been used successfully for almost a century in eastern Europe and the former Soviet Union. In the United States, phages have been used primarily for agricultural, food safety, industrial, and clinical diagnostic purposes.[57] Clinical trials in the United States and the European Union have had positive results. Since phages are prevalent in nature, concerns regarding their patentability have dampened pharmaceutical company interest. Nevertheless, some companies have managed to get around this challenge. For example, Gangagen holds patents for several whole-phage-based lethal agent systems that involve bacteriophages that have been genetically altered to improve their efficacy. Other phage patents involve parts of phages or purified phage lysins.[58]

Phage therapy presents other challenges. Phages have a limited spectrum of activity, so that physicians must identify the infecting microbe before prescribing therapy.[59] Better rapid diagnostic tests are needed to enable widespread use. Bacteria develop resistance to phages. One strategy to address this would be to use cocktail mixtures of three or more phages or to use phages in combination with antibiotics. Phages are often removed by patients' immune systems, limiting their usefulness in systemic infections; however, they have been used to treat septicemia (bloodstream infections) and pulmonary, gastrointestinal, urinary tract, and skin infections.[60]

As of March 11, 2015, a total of 29,501 R01 projects were in the NIH's Research Portfolio Online Reporting Tools system. An informal search of those mentioning "bacteriophage" or "phage" yielded 151 R01 projects. Of these, 23 were basic phage research projects and three were projects that focused on the potential antibacterial activity of phages.[61] One of these three projects examined lytic phage enzymes rather than the whole phage. Bacteriophages are very diverse, and whole phage families whose biology is still relatively unknown exist in nature. The NIH is expected to increase phage therapy research grants over the next year or two.[62]

Regulatory hurdles would have to be overcome to utilize bacteriocin or phage therapies. Currently, the FDA requires all molecules to undergo multiyear testing before receiving approval. For phages, the microbes might have already developed resistance before FDA approval. As with the influenza vaccine, which changes each year, the FDA would have to adjust its rules to exempt updated phage treatments from undergoing extensive, unnecessary clinical trials.[63]

Additional potential antibiotic therapies include molecules such as quorum-sensing inhibitors. After reaching a certain population density, bacteria produce and secrete signal molecules as a way to regulate group behavior. This is called "quorum sensing."[64] Bacteria that communicate through quorum sensing to produce biofilms are approximately 1,000 times as resistant to antibiotics as those that do not. Inhibitors that block quorum sensing constitute a potentially powerful strategy to prevent pathogenicity. For example, *P. aeruginosa* is a deadly pathogen that does not become virulent and produce a biofilm until its population size is large enough to overwhelm the host's immune system. A synthetic molecule, meta-bromo-thiolactone, prevented *P. aeruginosa* from producing pyocyanin, a virulence factor, and forming a biofilm.[65] Quorum-sensing inhibitors could provide important protective coatings for industrial membrane bioreactors in wastewater treatment facilities and for medical implants prone to biofilm contamination. They might also prove highly useful in preventing infections in aquaculture as well.[66]

The situation is not without hope. Although antibiotic resistance genes appear to be ancient and ubiquitous, advances in science and technology are expanding our understanding of the challenges. Efforts to develop new antibacterial therapeutics and diagnostics are growing. But these efforts will not negate the importance of using antibacterial drugs judiciously. Almost 50 percent of antibiotic use is considered inappropriate or unnecessary. Stringent stewardship programs for both humans and other animals need to be widely implemented to ensure appropriate antibiotic use.[67]

CHAPTER TEN

Conclusion

Medical and public health professionals fear that the era of antibiotics is coming to an end. Their concern is understandable. Bacterial resistance to antibiotics is reaching crisis levels, and not enough new therapeutics are replacing the old. This development could lead to severe consequences for the practice of modern medicine, as its foundation is built on the availability of safe and effective antibiotics. Without antibiotics, elective surgeries, cancer chemotherapies, organ transplants, autoimmune disease treatments, and other therapies might not be possible, because the risk of infection would be too high. Infections are becoming lethal, again.

At the same time, modern agriculture has become as dependent on antibiotics as modern medicine is. During the twentieth century, wars and droughts contributed to high food prices and, in some cases, food shortages. Many farmers went bankrupt and left farming. Modern agriculture evolved in response to these adversities to meet growing populations' demands for food, especially meat. Pigs and, to a lesser extent, poultry are the food animals that receive the most subtherapeutic antibiotics. They are also the most popular food animals in the world, accounting for more than 36 and 35 percent, respectively, of the meat consumed globally.[1] The advantages of raising pigs and poultry are that these animals are more efficient at converting feed into edible proteins and need less land and water than other terrestrial food animals such as beef cattle. Also, pigs and poultry produce less waste than dairy and beef cattle do. Of course, wastes from intensive livestock production facilities pollute the environment.[2] However, in defense of intensive agriculture, one study has shown that if separated from land spared for natural ecosystems, high-yield intensive agriculture conserves biodiversity better than agriculture that tries to integrate food production with conservation efforts.[3]

After exposure to antibiotics, humans and other animals produce feces that contain antibiotic residues, resistant microbes, and resistance genes. When spread on agricultural fields, they mix with soil bacteria, exchange genetic material, and alter the global resistome. Swine farm practices in China are particularly problematic in this regard. Manure runoff into streams and rivers and waste from aquaculture alter aquatic resistomes. Wild animals, especially birds, help spread resistance genes around the world.

The European Union's ban of subtherapeutic antibiotics in livestock has been promoted as an important strategy for addressing worsening antibiotic resistance. My analysis has found that the emergence of VRE in hospitals and on farms was the primary driver behind the antibiotic growth-promoter bans in Denmark and the European Union. These policy changes have had positive and possibly also negative consequences.

Clearly, banning avoparcin, the growth-promoting antibiotic related to vancomycin, was the right decision. Denmark's avoparcin ban led to 90 percent reductions of VRE in food animals. And while they did not have pre- and post-ban data to demonstrate a reduction of VRE carriage in healthy people, studies from Germany and the Netherlands did show a reduction.[4] Since reporting of VRE in livestock was voluntary, the European Union did not have enough VRE livestock data to assess the impact of the avoparcin ban across European countries. Unfortunately, this ban did not result in an overall reduction of VRE rates in hospitalized patients. Countries with high vancomycin use in humans were correlated with high VRE rates in hospitals. In Denmark, VRE rates in hospitalized patients increased in the years after the avoparcin ban. Genetic analyses provided a compelling explanation: VRE in hospitals differed genetically from VRE in food animals and healthy people; instead, they appeared genetically related to resistant enterococci isolated from dogs. These genomic findings of VRE, however, do not necessarily apply to other bacterial foodborne pathogens such as *Salmonella* species, *Campylobacter* species, and *Escherichia coli*.

Some countries have successfully reduced antibiotic use in livestock to levels lower than those in humans. In January 2015 the European Centre for Disease Prevention and Control (ECDC), the European Food Safety Authority (EFSA), and the European Medicines Agency (EMA) published a joint report analyzing antibiotic consumption and resistance in humans and food-producing animals.[5] Using 2012 data, the report indicated that in 26 EU or EEA countries, humans consumed a total of 116.4 mg/kg biomass of antibiotics (range: 56.7–175.8 mg/kg biomass), and food-producing animals con-sumed a total of 144.0 mg/kg biomass (range: 3.8–396.5 mg/kg biomass). But in 15 out of 26 countries, including Denmark, France, Norway, Sweden, and the United Kingdom, humans consumed more antibiotics in mg/kg biomass than food-producing animals. Food-producing animals consumed more tet-racyclines and aminoglycosides than humans, whereas humans consumed more penicillins, cephalosporins, and fluoroquinolones than food-producing animals.[6] The report did not examine changes in antibiotic consumption over time.[7]

The joint report found positive but borderline statistically significant as-sociations between tetracycline consumption in food-producing animals and tetracycline resistance in *Salmonella* species, *Campylobacter* species, and *E. coli* isolates from these animals. It did find a positive association between *Salmo-nella typhimurium* tetracycline resistance in human infections and tetracycline consumption in food-producing animals. The report found no association be-tween *E. coli* resistance to third-generation cephalosporins in humans and cephalosporin consumption in livestock, in contrast to the weakly positive correlation found in this book's analysis.[8] Unfortunately, the report did not include genomic data.

Danish data showed no decrease in pig-meat yield in the years immedi-ately after its antibiotic growth promoter ban, but Food and Agriculture Or-ganization (FAO) data suggests that the EU pig-meat yield, relative to the US yield, decreased approximately 3 percent, beginning in 2006, the year the growth-promoter ban commenced. If the 3 percent decrease in yield was due to the ban, then it might have cost the producers approximately $1.1 billion per year (in 2012 US dollars) in lost revenue. The cost to consumers is un-known; however, LABORSTA, the International Labor Organization, reports that retail prices of pork in some European countries have been generally higher than those in the United States.[9]

There was no evidence that EU poultry production was affected by the ban. But recall that the EU ban did not prohibit coccidiostat use because it is not possible to raise thousands or hundreds of thousands of birds together without these drugs. Coccidiostats do not have a counterpart in human med-icine, and low residues are not considered a risk to human health.[10]

In contrast to the European Union, the United States never approved avo-parcin, because of concerns about its carcinogenicity. With a few exceptions, VRE has not been detected in US food animals. Regardless, VRE has been a serious problem in US hospitals, most likely because of the extensive use of vancomycin in these settings. VRE appeared in US hospitals about a decade before becoming prevalent in European hospitals.

Tetracycline and ionophores (i.e., coccidiostats) are the most used antibiotics in US food animals. The United States also uses virginiamycin and tylosin as growth-promoting antibiotics. Not surprisingly, National Antimicrobial Resistance Monitoring System and National Animal Health Monitoring System data shows that nontyphoidal *Salmonella, Campylobacter jejuni,* and *E. coli* from chickens and pigs have high levels of tetracycline resistance. Nontyphoidal *Salmonella* and *E. coli* had zero and low levels of resistance to ciprofloxacin, respectively. Enterococcus from chickens, chicken meat, and pork chops showed high levels of quinupristin-dalfopristin resistance but zero resistance to vancomycin and linezolid.

For decades, the US Congress held hearings and requested reports seeking information regarding the risks of growth-promoting antibiotic use in livestock. Strong opposition by agriculture held off bans restricting their use. Agriculture succeeded in its lobbying efforts but ultimately lost public opinion and trust. With recommendations from the President's Council of Advisors on Science and Technology (PCAST) report, President Barack Obama issued an executive order in 2015 to combat antibiotic resistance and establish a national strategy to address the problem.[11] His proposed budget for fiscal year 2016 nearly doubles federal spending on antibiotic resistance, to more than $1.2 billion.[12] If approved by Congress, the increase in funding will help stimulate development of new antibiotics and rapid diagnostics, enhance surveillance of antibiotic resistance by incorporating a One Health approach, develop educational programs for physicians and veterinarians, and improve antibiotic stewardship in hospitals and farms, among other efforts. These initiatives will do much to mitigate the crisis. However, my investigation uncovered national and international issues that warrant further discussion.

1. *Veterinarians, farmers, and the pharmaceutical industry must be partners, not adversaries, in addressing antibiotic resistance.* In the United Kingdom, pharmaceutical companies and farmers were strongly opposed to the Swann Report's recommendations, which might explain why so little was accomplished after Parliament approved some of them. When the European Union passed the antibiotic growth-promoter ban in 2006, total antibiotic use in British livestock decreased only around 10 percent, even though growth-promoting antibiotic use fell to zero. In Sweden, pig farmers were committed to reducing

antibiotic use and improving animal welfare, which they did, even though some of them went out of business. Danish pig farmers were also committed to eliminating growth-promoting antibiotics but needed to use high doses of antibiotics when the animals got sick.

If the US Congress had mandated the cessation of subtherapeutic antibiotic use in livestock, farmers and pharmaceutical companies would have fought the ban and found ways to circumvent it. Instead, all 26 drug manufacturers have agreed to voluntarily phase out the production of medically important antibiotics for food-producing animals and phase in production of the remaining antibiotics for use under veterinarian oversight.[13] Medical and public health leaders might be unhappy with the slower, voluntary implementation of change, but it is arguably the most effective approach.

Unlike the European Union and the United States, where efforts to curtail antibiotic use in livestock are implemented or under way, respectively, other regions have different priorities. Rising incomes in low- and middle-income countries, such as India and China, are contributing to increasing demand for animal proteins, and livestock production in these countries is becoming increasingly intensive. Global consumption of antibiotics in food-animal production is expected to increase by an estimated 67 percent by 2030.[14]

In the United States, consumers are driving livestock producers to accommodate their demands for antibiotic-free meat. In 2014 around 5 percent of meat sold in the United States was antibiotic-free, but the proportion is rising rapidly. Large restaurant chains, such as McDonald's, are phasing in antibiotic-free meat to serve their customers.[15] It is unclear, however, what will happen to retail prices as more meat becomes antibiotic-free. Production costs for raising chickens without antibiotics are estimated to be 10 to 15 percent more than they are raised with antibiotics. In 2014 one retail food store sold antibiotic-free organic chicken breasts for $2.69 per pound while a generic store-brand chicken cost about $1.50 per pound. Some upscale retail stores sell organic, antibiotic-free chicken breasts for prices ranging from $8.99 to $10.00 per pound.[16] The affluent will have no problem affording antibiotic-free meat, but whether the poor will be able to afford more expensive meat is another matter.

2. *The management of human and animal waste must be improved.* Sanitation and hygiene are the foundation of public health, yet in many countries these straightforward interventions are not implemented. In the twenty-first century, people should not be openly defecating near their homes, and antibiotics

should not be relied on to treat diseases that should have been prevented by proper sanitation and hygiene. Approximately 2.6 billion people live without proper sanitation facilities. Even worse, 1 billion people practice open defecation, and of these, 82 percent live in 10 countries: China, Ethiopia, India, Indonesia, Mozambique, Nepal, Niger, Nigeria, Pakistan, and Sudan. In India almost 600 million people practice open defecation, representing approximately 60 percent of the 1 billion who openly defecate.[17] Not surprisingly, India stands out with some of the most resistant bacteria in the world. The combination of open defecation and abysmal sanitation contributes to India's severe disease burden and extensive misuse of antibiotics. Aside from building largely unused latrines, the Indian government has done very little to address these problems.

Poor sanitation and hygiene and contaminated drinking water lead to approximately 1.5 million preventable deaths from diarrheal diseases worldwide each year, mostly in children. In addition to causing diarrhea, poor sanitation provides breeding grounds for vector-borne diseases such as dengue. This viral disease has been mistakenly treated with antibiotics, another factor promoting antibiotic resistance.[18]

No nation should allow raw or minimally processed human or animal waste onto agricultural fields or other soils, or into bodies of water such as rivers, lakes, and oceans. This practice promotes the exchange of resistant genes, worsens the global resistome, and increases the risks of food- and waterborne diseases. Instead, sludge, the biomatter remaining after the removal of wastewater, should be disinfected before soil application. The contamination of wastewater and/or sludge with antibiotic-resistant microbes is not solely a problem of developing nations. Amos and colleagues developed predictive models of the environmental resistome by testing sites along the Thames River basin in the United Kingdom. They found that wastewater treatment plants were primarily responsible for introducing large numbers of antibiotic-resistant bacteria into the river. The size of the treatment plant, the type of treatment process, the season, and the rainfall level were factors that influenced the level of resistant bacteria in the environment.[19]

Much of the concern about antibiotic resistance has focused on the inappropriate use and overuse of antibiotics. This concern must be expanded to include human and animal waste containing resistant microbes, resistant genes, and antibiotic residues. More research is needed to understand the impact of treated and untreated waste on the global resistome and the costs necessary to treat it.

3. *Surveillance of resistant bacteria must include microbial genomes.* Without detailed genomic information, it is virtually impossible to understand the epidemiology of antibiotic-resistant microbes. VRE is a good example. Most scientists had assumed that VRE in hospitals emerged because of avoparcin use in livestock. The assumption seemed reasonable, since VRE had been isolated from farm animals and even from healthy people living in communities. Only after the genome was sequenced did it become clear that the hospital VRE population was genetically distinct from VRE in food animals and healthy humans. Antibiotic-resistance monitoring systems should include the genomes of VRE and other bacterial foodborne pathogens such as *Salmonella, Campylobacter,* and *E. coli.*

It is hard to develop effective policies with limited scientific information. Over the decades, scientific analyses of antibiotic resistance have focused on the plasmids that contained transmissible resistance genes shared between bacteria of the same and different species. This process allowed researchers to track the spread of resistance genes, but it did not provide them with enough information to determine the origin and genetic relationships between the resistant bacteria. Sequencing of bacterial genomes was needed. Before 2008 the cost of sequencing genomes was prohibitively expensive, around $10 million per genome. None of the government antibiotic-resistance surveillance systems included genome-sequencing data, because the technology was too expensive. Between 2009 and 2014, the cost decreased 95 percent. Research studies began to include genomic data. With time, the costs will likely decrease further, allowing the technology to become even more affordable for researchers and antibiotic-resistance surveillance program budgets. The PCAST report recommended that pathogen surveillance should be based on genome analysis.[20]

4. *Microbes and resistance genes from companion animals should be included in surveillance systems.* Genomic data suggested that enterococci isolated from dogs were genetically related to VRE in hospitals. Most of the attention on and concern about the source of antibiotic-resistant microbes has focused on food animals. The VRE example suggests that companion animals can play an important role in the transmission of antibiotic resistance. After all, they share people's homes and sometimes their food and beds.[21]

While methicillin-resistant *Staphylococcus aureus* (MRSA) is not considered a foodborne pathogen and has not been discussed in previous chapters of this book, its potential transmission by direct contact between animals and humans is worth noting. For example, Dr. Elizabeth Scott and colleagues swabbed the household surfaces of 35 randomly selected homes in the Boston area and found that half of them harbored MRSA. They discovered that cat owners were eight times more likely to have MRSA in their homes than people without cats.[22]

Companion animals have been largely ignored as potential sources of resistant microbes. There is no CDC for animals in general, and no surveillance system includes them. The intersection between companion animal and owner health is an area where a One Health approach would be important, requiring close collaboration between physicians and veterinarians in minimizing the risk of disease transmission between people and their pets. Such collaborations would be particularly important for companion-animal owners who are immunocompromised and depend on their pets for companionship.[23] The intersection of companion animal and owner health should be an integral component of clinical medicine, veterinary medicine, and public health.

5. *Human and animal microbiomes must be better understood to develop effective targeted therapies.* Scientific and technological advances have revealed that microbes influence the world in profound ways. The soils, the seas, and even the skies teem with them; they affect precipitation and possibly other weather events. The human microbiome project has found that healthy people's microbiomes differ considerably in the number and abundance of bacteria.[24] Human and other animal intestinal microbiomes contain approximately 100 trillion nonpathogenic bacteria.[25] Six to ten bacterial phyla, including *Proteobacteria, Actinobacteria, Bacteroidetes,* and *Firmicutes,* constitute the vast majority of the bacteria in these microbiomes. Alterations in human microbiota from widespread antibiotic use have been associated with diseases such as asthma, obesity, inflammatory bowel disease, psoriasis, and colorectal cancer.[26]

Finding safe alternatives to subtherapeutic antibiotics that are equally effective in improving feed utilization, promoting growth, and reducing mortality in livestock should be a priority. And indeed, an intense effort to find alternatives has been under way for more than two decades. Widely researched alternatives have included peptides, clay minerals, egg yolk antibodies, essential oils, enzymes, plant extracts, probiotics, lanthanoids (i.e., rare earth elements), copper, zinc, and others. Unfortunately, none have been as effective as antibiotics.[27]

6. *Clinicians should change the way they approach bacterial infections.* Reducing collateral damage to microbiomes will require more precision in diagnosing and treating infections. Time constraints and limited rapid diagnostic capabilities have forced clinicians to rely on broad-spectrum antibiotics that kill both beneficial and harmful bacteria. This approach will need to change as antibiotic resistance worsens and as science discovers more about the important roles microbes play in health.

Replenishing sick microbiomes is one strategy for treating infections. For example, fecal transplantations are increasingly being used to treat refractory *Clostridium difficile* infections, and cure rates of 90 percent are being reported. This treatment involves transferring feces from a healthy donor to the colon of a sick recipient. The first human fecal transplant was performed in 1958, but the medical community did not embrace the treatment until the late 1990s or the early years of the 2000s, after antibiotic resistance had become a serious problem. In contrast, veterinarians have been using fecal transplants for more than 100 years, infusing stools from healthy horses into the rectums of horses suffering from chronic diarrhea.[28]

In addition to new antibiotics, antibiotic alternatives are being developed, including bacteriocins, quorum-sensing inhibitors, and bacteriophages. Each has strengths and weaknesses. Bacteriophages require identifying the causative agent before therapy can be started, necessitating the need for accurate rapid diagnostic tests. Such tests would reduce inappropriate prescribing of antibiotics and the need for empiric therapy with broad-spectrum antibiotics. Standard diagnostic tests require at least 48 to 72 hours to identify the causative infecting bacteria, whereas rapid diagnostic tests can provide an answer within hours. Advances are being made. Hospital antibiotic stewardship programs are implementing rapid diagnostic tests to improve antibiotic use.[29] Ultimately, the goal is to improve both economic and clinical outcomes.

Although vaccines have not been previously discussed in this book and are not substitutes for antibiotics, they could reduce the need for antibiotics by preventing bacterial infections. In South Africa, four years after a pneumococcal conjugate vaccine was introduced in 2009, there was an 89 percent reduction in the rate of invasive pneumococcal disease in children, and rates of drug-resistant invasive pneumococcal disease had decreased by more than

50 percent. The state of Tennessee had similarly impressive reductions in antibiotic-resistant pneumococci rates within two years after the introduction of the pneumococcal conjugate vaccine.[30] The challenge with vaccines is diminishing public acceptance; vaccine-preventable diseases, such as pertussis and measles, are returning because parents are refusing to vaccinate their children. And as with antibiotics, pharmaceutical companies have been abandoning vaccines because they are not considered profitable.[31]

7. *Detailed antibiotic consumption data for humans and animals should be freely available on government websites; understanding why antibiotic consumption rates vary internationally and intranationally should be a priority.* The practice of medicine and veterinary medicine, including antibiotic prescribing behavior, varies from country to country.[32] Some countries, such as those in northern Europe, use antibiotics judiciously and sparingly; others, such as some of the southern European countries, use antibiotics much more freely.

Cultural, sociological, and economic factors that increase antibiotic use must be identified before they can be addressed.[33] In China, physicians and hospitals earned much of their revenue from prescribing and selling antibiotics before the Chinese government cracked down on their practices. Many countries continue to allow antibiotics to be sold over the counter as a substitute for health care. In Europe, the European Surveillance of Antimicrobial Consumption Network collects antibiotic consumption data in humans and makes it available on the ECDC website. While consumption rates for most antibiotics, including the cephalosporins, were freely available on the ECDC website, inexplicably, consumption rates specific to vancomycin were not. Vancomycin consumption rates were available on request, but the names of the countries could not be shared publicly. It is difficult to improve policies and practices if data is not openly available to highlight where problems exist. For example, India acknowledged its excessive use of antibiotics after a study was published documenting its high levels of consumption.[34] Acknowledging that a problem exists is the first step toward addressing it.

In the US, antibiotic consumption rates differ from state to state. However, the US government does not report human antibiotic consumption data. Instead, IMS Health, an information services and technology company, does.[35] This information is available for a price, hindering access for those with limited budgets.

In Europe, veterinary antibiotic sales data is freely available on the European Medicines Agency website. The first report, which covered the years 2005 to

2009, included only 9 countries. Since then, surveillance has expanded to include 26 EU or EEA countries.[36] As in human medicine, antibiotic sales varied between countries and did not necessarily correspond with the size of the livestock sector. In the United States, only since 2009 has the FDA been publishing veterinary antibiotic sales data for food animals.[37] The data is in aggregate form and does not specify which animals receive which drugs. Companion animals are not included in the reports.

Detailed regional-level data for human and veterinary medicine should be available, so that effective policies and guidelines can be developed. Recommendations for one region might not be relevant for another. With more precise data, policy recommendations could be tailored to high or low antibiotic-consuming regions, with regularly updated assessments.

Approximately 30 to 50 percent of antibiotics prescribed in US hospitals have been deemed inappropriate or unnecessary. Patient expectations, symptoms, duration of illness, and insufficient time for patient education all affect the likelihood that antibiotics will be prescribed.[38] In many countries, such as India and Pakistan, antibiotics are inappropriately prescribed, and patients inappropriately use them. Efforts are under way to change behavior. For example, in the United States in 1995, the CDC launched a National Campaign for Appropriate Antibiotic Use in the Community, which was renamed in 2003 Get Smart: Know When Antibiotics Work. The educational campaign focuses on upper-respiratory-tract infections, such as sinusitis, bronchitis, the common cold, and otitis media (i.e., ear infections), because these illnesses account for 75 percent of all the antibiotics prescribed by physicians in outpatient settings and are often considered inappropriate. The campaign has targeted both providers and patients.[39]

However, for veterinarians and pet owners, there are no government campaigns or guidelines for antibiotic prescribing and use. Other than the FDA's guidance 209 for industry, outlining the judicious use of antibiotics in food animals, no US federal agency has issued judicious antibiotic use guidelines for practicing large- or small-animal veterinarians. And, unlike the CDC's guidelines for infection control in outpatient and inpatient health care settings, there are no federal guidelines for infection-control measures in veterinary clinics or hospitals. Instead, the American Veterinary Medical Association (AVMA) issues judicious antibiotic use principles on its website, and the National Association of State Public Health Veterinarians (NASPHV) issues recommendations for infection control for veterinary practices on its website.[40]

8. *Governments must support early-career researchers who have novel, innovative ideas for basic science research.* As pharmaceutical companies disengaged from researching and developing new antibiotics in the early 1980s, the US government's approach to basic biomedical research became much more conservative in deciding who received grant funding. Instead of supporting young, innovative researchers starting out in their careers, the National Institutes of Health (NIH) preferred supporting older, established scientists with long track records. Many young scientists, unable to obtain research funding, left research entirely.[41]

Support for newly graduated PhDs with novel ideas should be a priority. Bruce Alberts, a professor in the Department of Biophysics and Biochemistry, University of California, San Francisco, and his colleagues recommended, among other things, that grants should focus on investigators at various stages in their careers to promote growth of new fields and increase the number of awards that emphasize originality and risk taking. Also, grant review panels should place higher priority on novelty, quality, and long-term objectives rather than on number of papers published and detailed descriptions of research methodologies.[42]

In addition to promoting young biomedical researchers, the government should increase support for young veterinary scientists. Since animals get many of the same diseases and infections as humans, a One Health research strategy could yield exciting, unexpected discoveries. Veterinary scientists approach diseases with unique perspectives that should be utilized. Instead, they are overlooked as principal investigators and collaborators in biomedical research. From 2008 to 2012, only 250 veterinarians out of 4,000 academic faculty at schools and colleges of veterinary medicine received NIH grant funding.[43]

9. *Pharmaceutical companies' interest in developing new therapeutics would increase if financial returns on investments were considered profitable.* Developing new drugs costs at least $1.2 billion spent over a decade. The dearth of new antibiotics has become so severe that one health policy expert suggested that wealthy nations (e.g., the United States, the European Union, and Japan) should jointly offer a $2 billion prize to the first five drug companies or universities that develop and get regulatory approval for a new class of antibiotics. But this flashy, one-time approach would not get at the root of the problem, which is long-standing pharmaceutical company disinterest because antibiotic research and development are not profitable. According to the 2014

PCAST report, pharmaceutical companies must have annual sales in the range of $400–600 million over 10 years to recoup their investments in antibiotic research and development.[44]

A few drug companies have made substantial investments in developing new antibiotics but face hurdles in making profits. For example, Durata Therapeutics developed dalbavancin, a new antibiotic indicated for bacterial skin infections, including MRSA. The drug is administered only twice, eight days apart, as 30-minute infusions; this regimen facilitates its use in outpatient settings. The company prefers an outpatient setting because Medicare pays for drugs administered in these settings separately at an average sales price with an added percentage, in contrast to inpatient hospital reimbursements, which are bundled in fixed diagnosis-related group payments. In an effort to increase inpatient reimbursements, the company submitted an application to the Centers for Medicare and Medicaid Services (CMS) for its drug to receive a new-technology add-on payment (NTAP) designation. NTAP is an effort by Congress to ensure that Medicare beneficiaries have timely access to new technologies, primarily devices, which would have been inadequately reimbursed under the existing government inpatient prospective payment system.[45] CMS denied Durata Therapeutic's application.[46] If recouping costs remains as difficult as it presently is, pharmaceutical companies will continue to shun developing and marketing new antibiotics.

The Generating Antibiotics Incentives Now (GAIN) Act of 2012 was an attempt by Congress to address the problem of inadequate reimbursement, but PCAST determined that it was unlikely to make any significant impact. The GAIN Act guaranteed an additional five years of market exclusivity for new antibiotics, but those five years would overlap with the patent protection of the drug, limiting any benefits for companies.[47] Ultimately, if societies want new antibiotics, they will have to come up with payment and/or subsidy strategies to make pharmaceutical companies' investments financially worthwhile.

10. *To increase international collaboration and cooperation, political leaders must agree on a global framework for antibiotic-related policies.* European Union policymakers based their decision to ban all antibiotic growth-promoting agents on the precautionary principle, a concept used for decision making when scientific uncertainty exists. The underlying premise of the precautionary principle is "to do no harm" or to make decisions using a "better safe than sorry" approach. The precautionary principle is often used when there

is concern about a drug's adverse impact on human health but cause-and-effect relationships have not been fully established.[48] The finding of VRE in European livestock drove the decision to ban not only avoparcin but also all antibiotic growth-promoting agents, even though the extent to which low-dose antibiotic use in livestock contributed to antibiotic resistance in humans was still under debate.

Critics of the precautionary principle argue that it provides no useful input in decision making. Instead, it is a rhetorical statement that allows political pressures to force government officials to defer long-term policy decisions. They contend that the precautionary principle is frequently used to prevent new technologies or products from being approved because they might cause harm. They assert that risk assessment should be used to make policy decisions because it has the most credibility. Rational, impartial decision making requires proper science-based assessments of benefits, costs, and risks.[49] The downside to this approach, however, is that the necessary data might not be available despite the need for immediate decisions.

The United States used the precautionary principle to withhold approval of avoparcin in the first place, for reasons unrelated to antibiotic resistance. The Delaney Clause required that the United States not approve the drug because enough data existed to raise concerns about cancer. This was not the first time when safety concerns prevented the United States from approving a drug that Europe allowed its population to use.[50] However, the United States does not necessarily use the precautionary principle in evaluating all new products.[51]

The European Union and the United States approached antibiotic resistance in different ways, but they continue to struggle with the issue because it is a global problem that requires global solutions. Antibiotic resistance has been compared to climate change. Both problems are global, intractable, and human-generated, and some have argued for the need for an independent international committee, analogous to the Intergovernmental Panel on Climate Change.[52]

The World Health Organization has published reports and dedicated a World Health Day to antibiotic resistance. On May 25, 2015, the 68th World Health Assembly met in Geneva, Switzerland, to endorse a draft resolution of a global action plan to address antimicrobial resistance. The draft resolution recognized the need for a One Health approach, and member states agreed to have national action plans aligned with the global action plan by May 2017.[53]

This draft resolution is an important first step, but it remains to be seen if member nations will have the commitment and wherewithal to implement national action plans.

If little progress is made by the two-year deadline, then a high-level political treaty, such as the 1997 Kyoto Protocol, to work cooperatively toward internationally agreed-upon targets might be needed.[54] A global framework for antimicrobial resistance should be developed, with interdisciplinary input from experts in medicine, public health, veterinary medicine, agriculture, and waste management, and other fields. The framework should include antibiotic consumption targets, sanitation and hygiene targets, manure management guidelines, harmonized antibiotic consumption and resistance surveillance guidelines, and public-outreach recommendations. All countries would commit to working toward the targets and adapt the guidelines to meet their needs.

In March 2015, the Obama administration released a National Action Plan to Combat Antibiotic Resistant Bacteria. This plan would serve as a five-year roadmap for implementing the policy recommendations of the PCAST report and would be consistent with the investments proposed in the president's FY 2016 budget. On April 3, 2015, an editorial in the *New York Times* criticized the newly released plan, stating that instead the United States should follow Denmark's lead and ban the use of medically important antibiotics for growth promotion in food-producing animals. The editorial stated that overall antibiotic use in Danish livestock fell by 50 percent after the ban. This is true, but the increase in therapeutic antibiotic use was not mentioned.[55] The politics continues.

History provides a cautionary tale regarding the fragility of the food supply. The use of growth-promoting antibiotics in livestock began during a time of high food prices after World War II. At that time, the national priority was food security: increase meat production and make food affordable. Since then, the priorities in the United States have changed. Food has been plentiful, and prices have been low. Antibiotic resistance has worsened, and demands to end the practice of using growth-promoting antibiotics in food-producing animals have increased. But worsening global climate disruptions such as severe droughts might bring back high food prices. Food security concerns might once again take precedence. And if food prices become too high, civil unrest can ensue.[56]

Efforts are under way to eliminate food-producing animals entirely by using protein substitutes beyond beans and other products. Growing artificial meat in laboratories is one option, but the technology is in its infancy. Edible insects are another option. Approximately 2 billion people in parts of Africa, Asia, and South America consume insects. In 2003 the UN Food and Agriculture Organization began the Edible Insects Program in recognition of insects' potential to provide protein to the estimated 9 billion people who will make up the world's population in 2050.[57] These protein alternatives would have to be appealing and palatable for people to accept them as part of their diets.

Ultimately, the politics of antimicrobial resistance involve food safety, food security, and sanitation. Everyone wants safe, affordable, nutritious food as well as safe, affordable, effective antibiotics. Sanitation and hygiene provide the necessary foundation for reducing disease burden and the need for antibiotics. Reaching the goal of having both organically raised antibiotic-free animal proteins and new effective antibiotics will cost money. Developed, affluent countries would be able to afford them, but poor, developing countries probably would not. The challenge for current and future political leaders is to figure out how to meet people's demands for animal proteins and antibiotics equitably, judiciously, and sustainably.

Acknowledgments

This book would not have been possible without my colleagues Bruce Kaplan, DVM; Tom Monath, MD; Jack Woodall, PhD; and Lisa Conti, DVM, MPH. Together, we manage the One Health Initiative website (www.onehealthinitiative .com), which serves as a global repository for all news and information pertaining to One Health, the concept that human, animal, and environmental health are linked. People from all over the world send us queries and comments about the concept.

On June 24, 2011, we received an e-mail from Dr. Ron Warner, a veterinarian with a master's degree in preventive medicine and a PhD in epidemiology, who was then the director of the Preventive Medicine Division in the Department of Family and Community Medicine, Texas Tech University Health Sciences Center. He wrote, "If multi-resistant human microbes evolve primarily in food animals, and foods of animal origin are the principal modes of transmission to humans, then we should expect to see (primarily) multi-resistant organisms isolated from foodborne outbreaks. I do not think that is what we see. What we primarily see in humans are multi-resistant organisms that are transmitted from person-to-person (e.g., multi-drug-resistant tuberculosis, methicillin-resistant *Staphylococcus aureus,* gonorrhea, streptococci, and others) . . . , not via the food chain." Dr. Warner brought to our attention the politics of antibiotic resistance and the blame game that has been going on for years between medicine and veterinary medicine.

I was intrigued by the controversy, because my interests include the politics of public health and the gaps that exist between human, animal, and environmental health. Dr. Warner's e-mail prompted me to begin a multiyear investigation of antibiotic use and resistance in humans and animals, primarily in Europe and the United States. Fortunately for me, virtually all government data was freely available online or by e-mail request.

I am grateful to Christopher Chyba, director of the Program on Science and Global Security (SGS) for his ongoing support. SGS is within Princeton University's Woodrow Wilson School of Public and International Affairs, and I am grateful to Dean Cecilia Rouse for the school's support of all of us within SGS.

Many people, including physicians, veterinarians, research scientists, historians, and government officials assisted me with my investigation: Frank M. Aarestrup, Yvonne Agerso, Markus Agito, Shukri Ahmed, Lis Alban, Eric Alm, Kristine Alpi, Camilla Alriksson, Sean Altekruse, Joseph F. Annelli, Karin Artursson, Marten Asp, Lennart Backstrom, Flemming Bager, Nicole Batey, Elena L. Behnke, Bjorn Bengtsson, Jeanine Bentley, Anne L. Berry, Tynesha Boomer, Douglas Bounds, Laura Bradbard, Eric J. Bush, David Byrne, Felipe C. Cabello, Richard Carnevale, Annemette Christensen, Annette Clauson, Jan Dahl, Spring Dahl, Gautam Dantas, Joann E. Donatiello, Catherine Dumartin, Bernadette M. Dunham, Gozke Duzer, Barry Eisenstein, Jimmie Enhall, Jorge Ferreira, Stephanie Fischer, Sheldon Garon, Jason Gill, Encarna Gimenez, Thomas M. Gomez, Christina Grecko, William Hahn, Charles Haley, Jonas Hammarstrand, Anette M. Hammerum, David Harvey, Eva Haxton, Birgitte Helwigh, Reba H. Higbee, Todd M. Hines, Christine Hoang, Birgitte Borck Hog, Jim Holding, David A. Hollander, (the late) H. Scott Hurd, Elizabeth Hutcheson, Amaney A. Jamal, Vibeke Frokjaer Jensen, Liz Kalina, Alan M. Kelly, Sue Kidd, Lonnie King, Moritz Klemm, Leonardo de Knegt, Helle Korsgaard, Annemarie Kuhns, Chris Lane, Sindre Langaas, Jorgen Nyberg Larsen, Maja Laursen, Dennis Lawler, Ramanan Laxminarayan, Stuart Levy, Barbro Liljequist, Joann M. Lindenmayer, Christian Lindeskov, Jonathan Lukkarinen, Alan E. Mann, Patrick McDermott, Gitte Lovschall Moller, Dominique Monnet, Prejit Nambiar, Joseph Nesme, Pia Nielsen, Asa Lannhard Oberg, Maureen Ogle, Bjorn Olsen, Dorthe C. Ostergaard, Suraj Pant, Rosa Peran, Marta Ponghellini, Nancy Pressman-Levy, Shelley Rankin, Hanne Rosenquist, Julie Rumsey, Jorgen Schlundt, Yvonne Siviter, Line Skjot-Rasmussen, Jan Slingenbergh, Anna Irene Vedel Sorensen, Kelley Squazzo, Gunnela Stahle, Cheryl Stroud, Christopher Teale, Susanne Maibom Teilgaard, Aude N. Teillant, John Threlfall, Janetta Top, Dora Navarro Torne, Ivar Vagsholm, Thomas Van Boeckel, Koen Van Dyck, Jacques Vianene, Carol Vreeland, Bruce A. Wagner, Ronald Warner, Martin Wierup, Christina Wikberger, and John T. Woolley.

Many thanks to Suzanne Flinchbaugh, formerly with Johns Hopkins University Press, for her interest and approval of my book proposal; to Jacqueline Wehmueller, executive editor at Johns Hopkins University Press; and to my editors Robin W. Coleman, Isla Hamilton-Short, Linda Benson, and Lois Crum.

Of course, I owe everything to my family, my husband, David Spergel, my children, Julian, Sarah, and Joshua, and my mother, Gladys S. Kahn, for their love, support, and willingness to hear about antibiotic resistance year after year. Finally, I am grateful to my golden retriever, Loki, who quietly slept in my office, keeping me company and occasionally forcing me to get up and take him for a walk.

Appendixes

Appendix A
Congressional Hearings and Activities on Subtherapeutic Use of Antibiotics in Livestock and Antibiotic Resistance

Date	Title	Bill Number / Committee (House/Senate)	Representative/Senator[1]
July 1945, 79th Congress	Penicillin Amendment to the Federal Food, Drug, and Cosmetic Act of 1938	N/A	N/A

Comments: Sec. 502 amended. Sec. 507 added. Federal Security Administrator (predecessor to FDA) must certify batches of any kind of penicillin for strength, quality, and purity, unless these requirements are not necessary to ensure safety and efficacy.[2]

Date	Title	Bill Number / Committee (House/Senate)	Representative/Senator[1]
March 1971, 92nd Congress	Hearing: Regulation of Food Additives and Medicated Animal Feeds	Government Operations (House)	Rep. L. H. Fountain (D-NC)

Comments: Focus on possible carcinogenic residues: DES, nitrates, nitrites, etc. Briefly mentioned antibiotic resistance.

Date	Title	Bill Number / Committee (House/Senate)	Representative/Senator[1]
June 1977, 95th Congress	GAO Report: Need to Establish Safety and Effectiveness of Antibiotics Used in Animal Feeds	Interstate and Foreign Commerce (House)	N/A

Comments: FDA allowed subtherapeutic use of antibiotics in livestock even though safety and effectiveness were not established.

Date	Title	Bill Number / Committee (House/Senate)	Representative/Senator[1]
Sept. 1977, 95th Congress	GAO Report: FDA's Regulation of Antibiotics Used in Animal Feeds	Interstate and Foreign Commerce (House)	N/A

Comments: FDA scientists determined that several antibiotics, including penicillin and tetracyclines, failed to meet safety criteria and created a hazard to human and animal health when used at low levels in animal feed. Many antibiotics had not been proved effective under approved conditions of use. Nevertheless, FDA continued to permit the use of subtherapeutic antibiotics in animal feeds.[3] Recommended that Secretary of HEW direct FDA commissioner to make a final determination of safety and effectiveness of antibiotics in animal feeds.

Date	Title	Bill Number / Committee (House/Senate)	Representative/Senator[1]
Sept. 1977, 95th Congress	Hearing: Antibiotics in Animal Feeds	Interstate and Foreign Commerce (House)	Rep. John E. Moss (D-CA)

Comments: Antibiotics in animal feed must be evaluated on three levels: human health hazards, animal health hazards, and antibiotic effectiveness.

Date/Congress	Title	Committee/Bill	Sponsor
Sept. 1977, 95th Congress	Hearing: Food Safety and Quality: Use of Antibiotics in Animal Feed	Agriculture, Nutrition, and Forestry (House)	Rep. Patrick J. Leahy (D-VT)

Comments: FDA statutory authority debated. Discussion on role of livestock and antibiotic resistance.

Date/Congress	Title	Committee/Bill	Sponsor
June 1979, 96th Congress	Office of Technology Assessment Report: Drugs in Livestock Feed	Requested by Senate Committee on Agriculture, Nutrition, and Forestry	Senator Herman E. Talmadge (D-GA)

Comments: Statutory authority limits FDA decisions to scientific evidence of safety and effectiveness—does not include economic considerations. Risks and benefits of subtherapeutic antibiotic use in livestock cannot be made using simple assessments.

Date/Congress	Title	Committee/Bill	Sponsor
May 1980, 96th Congress	Antibiotics Preservation Act	H.R. 7285	Rep. John Dingell, (D-MI)

Comments: Bill amended the Federal Food, Drug, and Cosmetic Act (FFDCA) to limit subtherapeutic antibiotic use in livestock. Died in committee.[4]

Date/Congress	Title	Committee/Bill	Sponsor
June 1980, 96th Congress	Hearing: Antibiotics in Animal Feed	Interstate and Foreign Commerce (House)	Rep. Henry A. Waxman (D-CA)

Comments: Antibiotics Preservation Act discussed. Proposed bill amended SEC 3. (a)(1) sec. 507 of the FFDCA (21 U.S.C. 357) to authorize FDA to restrict use of antibiotics, particularly penicillins and tetracyclines, in animal feed.

Date/Congress	Title	Committee/Bill	Sponsor
Oct. 1984, 98th Congress	Antibiotic Protection Act	H.R. 6370	Rep. James Weaver (D-OR)

Comments: Prohibited use of antibiotics certified for human use from being used in animal feed to promote growth. Referred to committee and died.[5]

Date/Congress	Title	Committee/Bill	Sponsor
Dec. 1984, 98th Congress	Hearing: Antibiotic Resistance	Science and Technology (House)	Rep. Albert Gore Jr. (D-TN)

Comments: Examined development of antibiotic resistance in humans and livestock. Debate over a 1984 *New England Journal of Medicine* study on links between subtherapeutic antibiotic use in livestock, beef, and human *Salmonella* infections. Suspected beef was never cultured.[6]

Appendix A *(continued)*

Date	Title	Bill Number / Committee (House/Senate)	Representative/Senator[1]
Jan. 1985, 99th Congress	Antibiotics Protection Act Reintroduced	H.R. 616	Rep. James Weaver (D-OR)

Comments: Weaver stated that proof of "smoking gun" is here and swift action is needed. He cited the 1984 *New England Journal of Medicine* article linking human *Salmonella* infections with beef. Bill died in committee.[7]

Feb. 1990, 101st Congress	Hearing: FDA's Regulation of Animal Drug Residues in Milk	Government Operations Committee (House)	Rep. Ted Weiss (D-NY)

Comments: Concern regarding the contamination of antibiotic residues in milk. Appropriate tests need to be developed and approved to monitor milk for possible residues.

Jan. 1992	GAO Report: FDA Needs Stronger Controls over the Approval Process for New Animal Drugs	Committee on Government Relations (House)	Rep. Ted Weiss (D-NY)

Comments: Under FFDCA, animal drug sponsors are responsible for demonstrating safety and effectiveness of products. Because of internal weaknesses, FDA is unable to ensure the accuracy and integrity of data submitted by sponsors.[8]

Feb. 1994, 103rd Congress	Animal Medicinal Drug Use Clarification Act	S. 340; H.R. 5056	Sen. Howell Heflin (D-AL), Rep. Charles Stenholm (D-TX)

Comments: Amended FFDCA to clarify the alternate uses of new animal drugs and new drugs intended for human use. Allowed veterinarians to prescribe extra-label uses of certain approved animal drugs and approved human drugs for animals under certain conditions.[9] Signed into law Oct. 22, 1994, becoming P.L. 103-396.[10]

Sept. 1995, 103rd Congress	OTA Report: Impacts of Antibiotic-Resistant Bacteria	Requested by House Committee on Energy and Commerce	N/A

Comments: Concluded that a risk exists. But direct evidence showing a connection between subtherapeutic antibiotic use in livestock and human death is difficult to obtain. In 1985 pigs were estimated to use the most antibiotics in livestock production: 68% of growth promotion and 63% of total antibiotic use.[11]

Oct. 1995, 104th Congress	Hearing: Emerging Infections: A Significant Threat to the Nation's Health	Labor and Human Resources (Senate)	Sen. Nancy L. Kassebaum (R-KS)

Comments: Cited 1992 Institute of Medicine report on Emerging Infectious Diseases. Hearing included expert testimony on ways legislation could address microbial threats. Antimicrobial resistance and the need for new antibiotics discussed.

Oct. 1996, 104th Congress	Animal Drug Availability Act	H.R. 2509; S. 773	Rep. Wayne Allard (R-CO), Sen. Nancy Kassebaum (R-KS)

Comments: Amended FFDCA to improve the process of approving and using animal drugs and medicated feeds, and for other purposes. Signed into law, P.L. 104-250, Oct. 1996.[12] Allowed flexibility in FDA process of evaluating and approving animal drugs. Created a new category of drugs: Veterinary Feed Directive drugs.[13]

Feb. 1999, 106th Congress	Hearing: Antimicrobial Resistance: Solutions for This Growing Public Health Threat	Health, Education, Labor, and Pensions (Senate)	Sen. Bill Frist (R-TN)

Comments: Antibiotic resistance compared to bioterrorism. Hearing focused on strengthening the public health infrastructure and improving surveillance to detect resistant microbes. The National Antimicrobial Resistance Monitoring Systems (NARMS), an interagency surveillance program, was described. An Interagency Task Force on Antimicrobial Resistance was recommended.[14]

April 1999	GAO Report: Food Safety: The Agricultural Use of Antibiotics and Its Implications for Human Health	Committee on Agriculture, Nutrition, and Forestry (Senate)	Senator Tom Harkin (D-IA)

Comments: Research linked use of antibiotics in livestock to emergence of human health pathogens: *Salmonella, Campylobacter,* and *E. coli.* But no comprehensive studies available that estimate the extent to which these resistant pathogens cause human illness and death.[15]

Date	Title	Bill Number/Committee (House/Senate)	Representative/Senator[1]
April 1999	GAO Report: Antimicrobial Resistance: Data to Assess Public Health Threat from Resistant Bacteria Are Limited	Committee on Health, Education, Labor, and Pensions (Senate) and Committee on Agriculture, Nutrition, and Forestry (Senate)	Sen. Edward Kennedy (D-MA), Sen. Tom Harkin (D-IA)

Comments: Found that full extent of problem of antimicrobial resistance remains unknown. Data on quantities of antimicrobials produced, used, and present in environment is not publicly available. Cited 1997 National Hospital Discharge Survey (NHDS), which found 43,000 patients diagnosed and treated for drug-resistant bacteria. In 1995 NHDS found 14,000 cases of VRE and 64,000 cases of ampicillin-resistant *E. coli.*[16]

Date	Title	Bill Number/Committee (House/Senate)	Representative/Senator[1]
Nov. 1999, 106th Congress	Preservation of Essential Antibiotics for Human Diseases Act	H.R. 3266	Rep. Sherrod Brown (D-OH)

Comments: Bill removed certain antibiotics essential to human health from being used subtherapeutically in livestock unless there was a reasonable certainty that no antimicrobial resistance would arise. Act amended the FFDCA. Died in subcommittee.[17]

Date	Title	Bill Number/Committee (House/Senate)	Representative/Senator[1]
June 2000, 106th Congress	Public Health Threats and Emergencies Act	H.R. 4964 and S. 2731	Rep. Richard Burr (R-NC), Sen. Bill Frist (R-TN)

Comments: Bill included provision to combat antimicrobial resistance. Established Antimicrobial Resistance Task Force, data collection, surveillance, promotion of research and development of new antibiotics. Became P.L. 106-505, title I; 114 Stat. 2315.

Date	Title	Bill Number/Committee (House/Senate)	Representative/Senator[1]
Sept. 2000, 106th Congress	Special Hearing: Antimicrobial Resistance	Appropriations (Senate)	Sen. Arlen Spector (R-PA)

Comments: Discussed public health action plan developed by interagency task force (FDA, CDC, NIH). Action plan included surveillance, prevention, education, and development of new antibiotics.

Date	Title	Bill Number/Committee (House/Senate)	Representative/Senator[1]
May 2001, 107th Congress	Antibiotic Resistance Prevention Act	H.R. 1771	Rep. Sherrod Brown (D-OH)

Comments: Provided funding for top-priority action items in the Interagency Action Plan. Died in a subcommittee.[18]

Date, Congress	Name	Bill Number	Sponsors
Oct. 2001, 107th Congress	Protecting the Food Supply from Bioterrorism Act	H.R. 3184; S. 1551	Rep. Rosa DeLauro (D-CT), Sen. Hilary Clinton (D-NY)

Comments: Amended FFDCA to protect the US food supply. Appropriated funding for surveillance of foodborne zoonotic and human diseases. Funded FDA's Food Safety Initiative. Not enacted.

March 2003, 108th Congress	Animal Drug User Fee Act	H.R. 1260; S. 313	Rep. Fred Upton (R-MI), Sen. John Ensign (R-NV)

Comments: Amended the FFDCA to establish a program of fees relating to animal drugs. Provided FDA with additional resources to evaluate new drug applications. Signed into law (P.L.108-130) Nov. 18, 2003.[19]

April 2004, 108th Congress	GAO Report: Federal Agencies Need to Better Focus Efforts to Address Risk to Humans from Antibiotic Use in Animals	Report to Senate Requesters	Sen. Olympia Snowe (R-ME), Sen. Tom Harkin (D-IA), Sen. Edward Kennedy (D-MA)

Comments: Many studies, especially genetic studies, found that use of antibiotics in animals posed risks to humans, but others found that health risks were minimal. Federal agencies lacked data on antibiotic use in animals. Secretaries of Agriculture and Health and Human Services should work together to develop and implement a plan to collect data.[20]

July 2004, 108th Congress	Project Bioshield	S. 15	Sen. Judd Gregg (R-NH)

Comments: Amended Public Health Service Act to provide protections and countermeasures against agents used in a terrorist attack. Created Strategic National Stockpile. Did not directly address antimicrobial resistance. Signed by President George W. Bush July 21, 2004, becoming P.L. 108-276.[21]

Dec. 2006, 109th Congress	Pandemic and All-Hazards Preparedness Act	S. 3678	Sen. Richard Burr (R-NC)

Comments: Ensured pandemic and biodefense vaccine and drug development. Biomedical Advanced Research and Development Authority (BARDA) established; responsible for antibiotics as part of Project BioShield mandate. Bill signed by President George W. Bush, Dec. 19, 2006, becoming P.L. 109-417.[22]

Appendix A (continued)

Date	Title	Bill Number / Committee (House/Senate)	Representative/Senator[1]
Feb. 2007, 110th Congress	Preservation of Antibiotics for Medical Treatment	H.R. 962	Rep. Louise Slaughter (D-NY)

Comments: Bill targeted subtherapeutic antibiotic use in livestock. Cited the 1999 EU ban of medically important antibiotics in livestock for growth promotion, stating that those countries experienced no significant impact on animal health or productivity; levels of resistant bacteria declined sharply. Died in committee.

Date	Title	Bill Number / Committee (House/Senate)	Representative/Senator[1]
Sept. 2007, 110th Congress	Food and Drug Administration Amendments Act (FDAAA)	H.R. 3580	Rep. John Dingell (D-MI)

Comments: Bill included language to encourage new antibiotic development. President George W. Bush signed it into law.[23]

Date	Title	Bill Number / Committee (House/Senate)	Representative/Senator[1]
Sept. 2007, 110th Congress	Strategies to Address Antimicrobial Resistance Act	H.R. 3697; S. 2313	Rep. Jim Matheson (D-UT), Sen. Sherrod Brown (D-OH)

Comments: Amended Public Health Service Act to create an Antimicrobial Resistance Task Force to create a strategic research plan, enhancing efforts against antimicrobial resistance. Referred to committee.[24] Bill created government infrastructure to collect data, coordinate research, and collect surveillance data to address problem. Not enacted.

Date	Title	Bill Number / Committee (House/Senate)	Representative/Senator[1]
June 2008, 110th Congress	Hearing: Emergence of the Superbug: Antimicrobial Resistance in the US	Health, Education, Labor, and Pensions (Senate)	Sen. Edward Kennedy (D-MA)

Comments: Human and animal health experts debated the role of subtherapeutic antibiotics in livestock as a cause of antibiotic resistance. Discussed how to get pharmaceutical companies interested in developing new antibiotics.

Date	Title	Bill Number / Committee (House/Senate)	Representative/Senator[1]
July 2008, 110th Congress	Animal Drug User Fee Amendments	H.R. 6432	Rep. Frank Pallone Jr. (D-NJ)

Comments: Extended the Animal Drug User Fee Act of 2003. Signed into law, becoming P.L. 110-316.[25] Strengthened FDA's ability to collect animal antibiotic distribution data.[26]

Date	Title	Bill Number / Committee (House/Senate)	Representative/Senator[1]
May 2009, 111th Congress	Strategies to Address Antimicrobial Resistance Act	H.R. 2400	Rep. Jim Matheson (D-UT)

Comments: Reintroduced and referred to committee, where it died.

Date	Title	Bill/Type	Sponsor
July 2009, 111th Congress	Preservation of Antibiotics for Medical Treatment	H.R. 1549	Rep. Louise Slaughter (D-NY)

Comments: Reintroduced bill amended Sec. 201 of the FFDCA (21 U.S.C. 321) for a phased elimination of subtherapeutic antibiotic use in animals. Would withdraw approval of use of nontherapeutic antibiotics in food animals. Bill died.

Dec. 2009, 111th Congress	Speech: Antibiotics in Animal Agriculture	House	Rep. Leonard Boswell (D-IA)

Comments: Given permission to speak for one minute before House. Stated that animal agriculture was under attack. The industry used antibiotics responsibly. Banning antibiotic use would penalize an industry without appropriate data to back claims of harm. A ban would have detrimental effects on livestock and public health.

April 2010, 111th Congress	Hearing: Antibiotic Resistance and Threat to Public Health (1st in series of 3 hearings)	Energy and Commerce (House)	Rep. Frank Pallone Jr. (D-NJ)

Comments: Highlighted problems associated with antibiotic-resistant bacteria and the work being done to address them. Rep. Joseph Pitts, Pennsylvania, stated, "The National Institutes of Allergy and Infectious Diseases acknowledges there is a debate about the public health impact" of antibiotic use in animal agriculture, particularly in animal feed.[27]

June 2010, 111th Congress	Hearing: Promoting the Development of Antibiotics and Ensuring Judicious Use in Humans (2nd in series of 3 hearings)	Energy and Commerce (House)	Rep. Frank Pallone Jr. (D-NJ)

Comments: Focused on human use of antibiotics. The more antibiotics are used, the less effective they become—not a good business model for companies to develop new antibiotics. Resistance has added costs to the nation's health care bill. FDAAA of 2007 called on FDA to assess if Orphan Drug Act could be applied to antibiotics. FDA concluded "no."[28]

July 2010, 111th Congress	Hearing: Antibiotic Resistance and the Use of Antibiotics in Animal Agriculture (3rd in series of 3 hearings)	Energy and Commerce (House)	Rep. Frank Pallone, Jr. (D-NJ)

Comments: Pallone stated, "The challenge will be to not move into public policy until we have verifiable peer-reviewed science to address this issue." The Infectious Disease Society of America and the Pew Charitable Trusts debate the role of antibiotics in food animals with the AVMA and the veterinary medical profession: "precautionary principle" versus "risk assessment."

Appendix A (continued)

Date	Title	Bill Number/Committee (House/Senate)	Representative/Senator[1]
Sept. 2010, 111th Congress	Generating Antibiotic Incentives Now (GAIN) Act	H.R. 6331	Rep. Phil Gingrey, MD (R-GA)

Comments: Amended the FFDCA by including an extension of exclusivity period for new qualified infectious disease products.[29] Died in committee.

March 2011, 112th Congress	Preservation of Antibiotics for Medical Treatment Act	H.R. 965; S. 1211	Rep. Louise Slaughter (D-NY), Sen. Dianne Feinstein (D-CA)

Comments: Reintroduced bill from previous session. Died in committee.

June 2011	GAO Report: Antibiotic Resistance: Data Gaps Remain despite HHS Taking Steps to Improve Monitoring	Agriculture (House)	Rep. Frank D. Lucas (R-OK), Rep. Collin Peterson (D-MN)

Comments: Federal agencies could use sales data as an estimate of antibiotic production in humans. Better data could help policymakers determine what proportion of human antibiotic use contributes to resistance.[30]

June 2011, 112th Congress	Generating Antibiotic Incentives Now (GAIN) Act of 2011	H.R. 2182; S. 1734	Rep. Phil Gingrey, MD (R-GA), Sen. Richard Blumenthal (D-CT)

Comments: Essentially same bill as introduced in 2010, but with more detail regarding exclusivity of new infectious disease product. Died in committee.[31]

June 2011, 112th Congress	National Sustainable Offshore Aquaculture Act	H.R. 2373	Rep. Lois Capps (D-CA)

Comments: Reintroduced after failed 2009 introduction. Established a regulatory and research program for sustainable offshore aquaculture; prohibited use of antibiotics except for treatment of disease and after consultation with commissioner of FDA. Died in committee.[32]

Date	Title	Bill/Committee	Sponsor
Sept. 2011	GAO Report: Agencies Have Made Limited Progress Addressing Antibiotic Use in Animals	Rules (House)	Rep. Louise Slaughter (D-NY)

Comments: HHS and USDA data on antibiotic use in livestock lacks crucial details needed to examine trends and determine relationship between use and resistance.[33]

Sept. 2011, 112th Congress	Foodborne Illness Reduction Act	S. 1529	Senator Kirsten Gillibrand (D-NY)

Comments: Required USDA to protect against foodborne illnesses by establishing a more effective, preventive food safety system administered by the USDA Food Safety and Inspection Service. Included monitoring for antimicrobial-resistant pathogens.[34] Not enacted.

Jan. 2012	GAO Report: FDA Needs to Do More to Ensure That Drug Labels Contain Up-to-Date Information	Committee on Health, Education, Labor, and Pensions (Senate); Committee on Energy and Commerce (House)	Sen. Tom Harkin (D-IA), Sen. Michael Enzi (R-WY), Rep. Fred Upton (R-MI), Rep. Henry Waxman (D-CA)

Comments: FDA has had difficulty ensuring that antibiotic producers give up-to-date information (i.e., "breakpoint") on bacterial resistance on drug labels. The FDAAA provisions to promote antibiotic innovation have not been successful.[35]

March 2012, 112th Congress	Hearing: FDA User Fees 2012: Issues Related to Accelerated Approval, Medical Gas, Antibiotic Development, and Downstream Pharmaceutical Supply Chain	Energy and Commerce (House)	Rep. Joseph Pitts (R-PA)

Comments: Hearing focused on issues related to FDA user-fee program. Addressed lack of new antibiotics and ways Congress and FDA could increase incentives for new antibiotic development.

May 2012, 112th Congress	Food and Drug Administration Safety and Innovation	S. 3187	Sen. Thomas Harkin (D-IA)

Comments: Bill incorporated GAIN Act with extension of exclusivity period for new antibiotics. Signed by President Obama in July 2012, becoming P.L. 112-144.[36]

Appendix A *(continued)*

Date	Title	Bill Number / Committee (House/Senate)	Representative/Senator[1]
Feb. 2013	Delivering Antimicrobial Transparency in Animals Act	H.R. 820	Rep. Henry Waxman (D-CA)
Comments: Amended FFDCA to enhance reporting requirements of antimicrobial drugs in livestock. Cited P.L. 110-316, which requires FDA to collect sales data from producers of drugs. Referred to committee.[37]			
March 2013, 113th Congress	Preservation of Antibiotics for Medical Treatment Act	H.R. 1150	Rep. Louise Slaughter (D-NY)
Comments: Reintroduced bill. Referred to committee.			
June 2013, 113th Congress	Strategies to Address Antimicrobial Resistance Act	H.R. 2285; S. 2236	Rep. Jim Matheson (D-UT), Sen. Sherrod Brown (D-OH)
Comments: Reintroduced and referred to committee.			
June 2013, 113th Congress	Preventing Antibiotic Resistance Act	S. 1256	Sen. Dianne Feinstein (D-CA)
Comments: Mandated a phased elimination of nontherapeutic use in animals of medically important antibiotics.[38]			
Sept. 2013, 113th Congress	Safe Meat and Poultry Act	S. 1502	Sen. Kirsten Gillibrand (D-NY)
Comments: Included provisions for state-of-the-art DNA matching system and epidemiology system dedicated to identifying foodborne illness. Required analysis of incidence of antimicrobial drug resistance as pertaining to the food supply and developed new methods to reduce transmission.[39]			

Appendix B

FDA Actions Regarding Subtherapeutic Antibiotics in Livestock

Date	FDA Action	Comments
1951	Penicillin, streptomycin, chloramphenicol, and other antibiotics are approved for use in animal feed.	Exempted from requirements of secs. 502 (1) and 507 of the 1945 Penicillin Amendment.[1]
1966	Ad hoc Committee on the Veterinary Medical and Nonmedical Uses of Antibiotics.[2]	Recommended that sponsors of drugs containing antibiotics intended for livestock should submit data to determine whether residues are present in food from the treated animals.
April 1970	Task Force Report: The Use of Antibiotics in Animal Feed.	Report recommended that certain antimicrobial drugs used in human medicine should not be used for growth promotion and should be limited to short-term therapeutic use by a veterinarian's prescription.[3]
Jan. 1972	Task Force Report.	Noted that the feeding of certain antibiotics to animals may lead to resistant bacteria in humans. The safety and efficacy of long-term use of subtherapeutic antibiotics had not been demonstrated.[4]
April 1973	Published final rule that established 21 CFR 135.109: Antibiotic and sulfonamide drugs in the feed of animals (redesignated in 1974 as sec. 558.15). In September 1973, section was amended to include nitrofurans (38 FR 23942).[5]	FDA wrote regulations implementing task force recommendations, stating that approval of subtherapeutic antibiotics in animal feeds would be revoked in two years unless manufacturers submitted data proving safety and efficacy.[6] Regulations were not implemented.
June 1975	Established an Antibiotics in Animal Feeds Subcommittee of its National Advisory Food and Drug Committee (NAFDC).[7]	Subcommittee was meant to be a policy advisory committee. It reviewed data on penicillin, tetracyclines, and sulfaquinoxaline.
Jan. 1977		Subcommittee recommended that penicillin growth-promotion use be discontinued and tetracycline growth-promotion use be discontinued when effective substitutes become available. Approved continued use of sulfaquinoxaline, if limited to periods when threat of animal disease was greatest.[8]

Appendix B (continued)

Date	FDA Action	Comments
Jan. 1977		NAFDC accepted penicillin and sulfaquinoxaline recommendations but rejected tetracycline recommendations. One committee member, the president of Farr Farms, a Colorado feedlot, took an active role in rejecting initial recommendation to discontinue tetracycline use. Controversy over conflict of interest ensued.[9]
April 15, 1977	FDA announced plans to restrict use of penicillin, tetracyclines, and sulfaquinoxaline in animal feeds based on GAO recommendation.	Rejected recommendations made by NAFDC. FDA determined that only three antibiotics met all safety criteria for low-level use: bacitracin, flavomycin, and oleandomycin.[10]
August 30, 1977	FDA published in *Federal Register* a Notice of Opportunity for Hearing proposing to withdraw approval for all animal feed uses of penicillin and certain uses of tetracyclines.[11]	Proposal was criticized because of insufficient epidemiological evidence that bacteria of animal origin caused serious illness in humans and failed to be enacted by congressional order. FDA subsequently contracted with National Academy of Sciences to conduct safety study of antimicrobial use in food animals.[12]
1984	Seattle–King County Study: "Surveillance of the Flow of *Salmonella* and *Campylobacter* in a Community."	FDA contracted Seattle–King County Health Department to study the relationship between *Salmonella* species and *Campylobacter jejuni* in foods of animal origin and human disease. Study found that *C. jejuni* caused more human enteritis than *Salmonella* and that it occurred via consumption of poultry products. Plasmid-mediated tetracycline resistance was also transmitted from food to humans.[13]
1998	FDA Task Force on Antimicrobial Resistance established.	Developed key priorities for the agency given limited resources.
Jan. 1999	FDA published concept paper, "Proposed Framework for Evaluating and Assuring the Human Safety of the Microbial Effects of Antimicrobial New Animal Drugs Intended for Use in Food-Producing Animals."	Proposed strategies for managing potential risks associated with antibiotic use in livestock.

Date	Document	Description
June 1999	Public Health Action Plan to Combat Antimicrobial Resistance.	Interagency Task Force on Antimicrobial Resistance established to develop a blueprint for specific, coordinated efforts between federal agencies to address antimicrobial resistance. Lacks high-level, centralized leadership to measure progress and accountability.[14]
Oct. 1999	FDA Task Force Report published.	Focused on four key areas: respond to current threats, facilitate product development, facilitate safe and effective antibiotic use, and coordinate scientific response to antimicrobial resistance.
Jan. 2001	Federal Interagency Task Force (e.g., FDA, NIH, CDC, among others) released action plan to address antimicrobial resistance.	Recommended improving antimicrobial surveillance, prevention and control, research, and product development.[15]
Oct. 2003	Guidance for Industry #152: Evaluating the Safety of Antimicrobial New Animal Drugs with regard to their microbiological effects on bacteria of human health concern.[16]	Drugs must be safe and effective for food animals and safe with regard for human health. Outlined a risk-assessment approach for evaluating the microbial food safety of new antimicrobials. Risk-analysis process was based on process described by the Office International des Epizooties Ad Hoc Group on Antimicrobial Resistance;[17] included hazard identification, risk assessment, and risk management, providing a qualitative indication of the potential human health risk posed by the new veterinary antimicrobial drug. Appendix A of the document ranks antimicrobials into three groups depending on their importance in human medicine: critically important, highly important, and important. Appendix A to be periodically reassessed and updated.[18]
April 2004	Guidance for Industry #144: Pre-Approval Information for Registration of New Veterinary Medicinal Products for Food-Producing Animals with Respect to Antimicrobial Resistance	Harmonized technical guidelines (to be used by regulatory bodies in the EU, Japan, and the United States) for the approval of therapeutic antimicrobial veterinary medical products. Sponsors should include in their new drug applications data on antimicrobial resistance mechanisms, genetics, and occurrence and rate of transfer of resistance genes, among other information.[19]

Appendix B (continued)

Date	FDA Action	Comments
July 2005	FDA bans use of enrofloxacin (a fluoroquinolone) for treating bacterial infections in poultry.	Agency cited scientific evidence demonstrating that fluoroquinolone resistance emerges in *Campylobacter*, which causes foodborne illnesses.[20]
March 2010	Proposed rule change regarding Veterinary Feed Directive (VFD) in *Federal Register*.[21]	Review of VFD regulations, initially effective Jan. 8, 2001, relating to distribution and use of VFD drugs and animal feeds containing drugs. Public comment solicited.
June 2010	Released draft guidance, "The Judicious Use of Medically Important Antimicrobial Drugs in Food-Producing Animals."	Informed public of FDA's thinking on the use of medically important antimicrobial drugs in livestock.
July 2010	Cosponsored public workshop with IDSA and NIAID, "Issues in Antibacterial Resistance and Device and Drug Development"	Approximately 60–70% of all antimicrobials are used in outpatient settings. About 50% of the antibiotics prescribed in outpatient settings are unnecessary. Most common diagnoses receiving antibiotics: otitis media, pharyngitis, sinusitis, bronchitis, and common cold. Top three reasons for provider overprescribing: patient demand, provider fear of missing a bacterial infection, fear of litigation. Rapid diagnostics will play an important role in reducing unnecessary antibiotic use.[22] Unlike Europe, the United States does not have antimicrobial use data available, and there is no systematic way to collect it. Also, many US hospitals are outsourcing their microbiology labs, reducing the availability of minimal inhibitory concentration resistance data.[23] CDC's antimicrobial resistance budget was only $17 million with a proposed 50% cut.[24]

April 2012	Guidance for Industry #209. The Judicious Use of Medically Important Antimicrobial Drugs in Food-Producing Animals.[25]	FDA developed a framework for the voluntary adoption of practices to limit medically important antimicrobials for use in food-producing animals. Antibiotics should be administered only when the animals' health is at stake. And the drugs should be given only through the oversight of veterinary medical professionals. Guidelines not legally enforceable.[26]
Dec. 2013	Guidance for Industry #213. New Animal Drugs and New Animal Drug Combination Products Administered in or on Medicated Feed or Drinking Water of Food-Producing Animals: Recommendations for Drug Sponsors for Voluntarily Aligning Product Use Conditions with GFI #209.[27]	FDA does not consider the use of medically important antibiotics in food-producing animals for growth promotion to be judicious use. However, it does consider antibiotic treatments, controls, or preventions targeted against specific diseases to be judicious use. FDA expected drug sponsors to voluntarily comply with guidelines. New animal drugs are approved in one of three marketing categories: over-the-counter, veterinary prescription, veterinary feed directive. FDA plans three-year phase-in for animal drug sponsors to voluntarily make changes to management and business practices.[28]

US National Academy of Sciences/National Research Council/Institute of Medicine Reports

Date	Title	Comments
1966	NAS report: "A Historical Survey of Animal Disease Morbidity and Mortality Reporting"	Subcommittee on Methods and Procedures for Reporting Animal Morbidity and Mortality of the Committee on Animal Health subsequently recommended a nationwide surveillance system for animal health. Report led to a special panel with task of designing such a system.[1]
June 1969	NAS Committee on Salmonella	Recommended that only minimal amounts of antibiotics be used in feed and water to promote growth.[2]
1974	NRC: A Nationwide System for Animal Health Surveillance	Special panel with task of designing a nationwide animal health surveillance system publishes report. Recommends that a "center" be established as a national focal point for collecting, compiling, analyzing, and disseminating epidemiological data and costs of animal diseases.[3]
1980	NRC: The Effects on Human Health of Subtherapeutic Use of Antimicrobials in Animal Feeds	Not possible to do a comprehensive epidemiological study of human health risks from subtherapeutic antibiotic use in livestock. Impossible to determine antibiotic history from a piece of meat.[4]
1988	IOM: Human Health Risks with the Subtherapeutic Use of Penicillin or Tetracyclines in Animal Feed	By FDA request, IOM committee developed a risk-analysis model including annual numbers of reported cases of specific infections, fraction of cases due to bacterial resistance, mortality rates, and fractions of deaths associated with strains of farm animals. Salmonella was selected for risk model because of considerable data reported over many years. Did not address cost-benefit issues. Found indirect, circumstantial evidence but unable to find data directly linking subtherapeutic use in livestock with human illness.[5] Recommended further study.
1992	IOM: Emerging Infections: Microbial Threats to Health in the United States	Report focuses primarily on emerging viral diseases and the need for greater vaccine development and public health capabilities. Drug development should not be left entirely to free enterprise but rather be an integrated national process. Antibiotic development should be publicly financed and approval should be expedited. Human clinicians, veterinarians, and users in agriculture should be educated on proper use.[6]

Year	Title	Description
1998	IOM: Antimicrobial Resistance: Issues and Options: Workshop Report	There has been a lack of data, particularly data from veterinary reference labs. An ecological understanding of conditions that enhance resistance would help. USDA, AVMA, FDA, and livestock producers should work together to increase understanding on this issue.[7] Recommended a National Antimicrobial Surveillance System in humans and animals.[8]
1999	NRC: The Use of Drugs in Food Animals: Benefits and Risks	A joint effort between Panel on Animal Health, Food Safety, and Public Health and Institute of Medicine evaluated risks and benefits of drug use in livestock industry. Concluded that a link exists between antibiotic use in livestock and human disease, but incidence is very low.[9]
2003	IOM: Microbial Threats to Health: Emergence, Detection, and Response	Recommended, among other things, "that FDA should ban the use of antimicrobials for growth promotion in animals if those classes of antimicrobials are also used in humans."[10]
2010	IOM: Antibiotic Resistance: Implications for Global Health and Novel Intervention Strategies: Workshop Summary	Reviewed history of antibiotic development and subsequent microbial resistance. Antibiotic usage likened to "tragedy of the commons" for inappropriate personal gain at the expense of societal need.[11]
2012	IOM: Improving Food Safety Through a One Health Approach	Cites international legal framework involved in control of foodborne antimicrobial resistance: Codex Alimentarius Commission under WHO and FAO recommendations. Regulatory authorities should mandate that all antibiotics be prescription only. Surveillance systems to monitor antibiotic use and resistance should be established in all countries. Professional organizations should develop clinical practice guidelines for antibiotic use.[12]
2014	NRC: Technical Challenges in Antibiotic Discovery and Development: A Workshop Summary	Since 1987 no new antibiotics have been discovered. Three organisms pose the greatest public health urgency: Carbapenem-resistant *Enterobacteriaceae*, resistant *Neisseria gonorrhea*, and *Clostridium difficile*. Genomics, proteomics, and other novel areas are increasingly being used to identify new drug targets beyond the resistant factors.[13]

Notes

CHAPTER ONE: The Politics

1. In this book, the term "nontherapeutic antibiotics" is used synonymously with "subtherapeutic antibiotics" and "growth-promoting antibiotics."

2. Stephanie Strom, "Report on U.S. Meat Sounds Alarm on Resistant Bacteria." *New York Times,* April 16, 2013, www.nytimes.com/2013/04/17/business/report-on-us-meat-sounds -alarm-on-superbugs.html.

3. In the United States, the FDA Center for Veterinary Medicine considers any extended use, beyond two weeks, of antibiotics in feed at 200 g/ton or less as "subtherapeutic" if used for disease prevention or growth promotion. Institute of Medicine, *Human Health Risks with the Subtherapeutic Use of Penicillin or Tetracyclines in Animal Feed: Report of a Study* (Washington, DC: National Academies Press, 1989), p. iii, www.fda.gov/ohrms/dockets/dailys/03/Aug03 /081403/03n-0324-bkg0001-05-tab-4-01-vol2.pdf.

4. American Farm Bureau Federation, "Preserving Antibiotics Access," www.fb.org/issues /docs/antibiotics12.pdf.

5. S. B. Levy, *The Antibiotic Paradox: How Miracle Drugs Are Destroying the Miracle* (New York: Plenum Press, 1992), p. 156.

6. Strom, "Report Sounds Alarm." NARMS monitors the trends of antimicrobial resistance in four key bacteria: *Salmonella, Campylobacter, Enterococcus,* and *Escherichia coli.* The NARMS 2011 Retail Meat Report found over nine years (2002–11) a two-and-a-half-fold increase of multi-drug resistance in *Salmonella* in poultry. Multi-drug resistance remained rare in *Campylobacter,* but from 2007 to 2011, resistance to gentamicin increased twenty-five-fold. For *Enterococcus* and *E. coli,* resistance varied depending on the antibiotic. U.S. Department of Health and Human Services, *National Antimicrobial Resistance Monitoring System (NARMS) 2011 Retail Meat Report,* www.fda.gov/AnimalVeterinary/SafetyHealth/AntimicrobialResistance/Nat ionalAntimicrobialResistanceMonitoringSystem/ucm334828.htm.

7. Environmental Working Group, "Superbugs Invade American Supermarkets," April 2013, http://static.ewg.org/reports/2013/meateaters/ewg_meat_and_antibiotics_report2013 .pdf.

8. Bernadette Dunham, "Resistant Bacteria in Meat," letter to the editor, *New York Times,* April 23, 2013, www.nytimes.com/2013/04/24/opinion/resistant-bacteria-in-meat.html?_r=0.

9. Louise M. Slaughter, "Limiting Antibiotics in Animals," letter to the editor, *New York Times,* April 29, 2013, www.nytimes.com/2013/04/30/opinion/limiting-antibiotics-in-animals .html?emc=eta1&_r=0. In this letter, Congresswoman Slaughter also wrote, "Evidence on this is so clear that the American Medical Association, the World Health Organization, the Union of Concerned Scientists and 450 groups support my legislation to save eight classes of antibiotics for human health."

10. CDC 2011 Estimates, www.cdc.gov/foodborneburden/PDFs/FACTSHEET_A_FINDINGS _updated4-13.pdf.

11. C. Kabera, personal communication; FDA, The National Antimicrobial Resistance Monitoring System, Reports and Data, www.fda.gov/AnimalVeterinary/SafetyHealth/Anti microbialResistance/NationalAntimicrobialResistanceMonitoringSystem/ucm059103 .htm.

12. V. O. Stockwell and B. Duffy, "Use of Antibiotics in Plant Agriculture." *Scientific and Technical Review of the Office International des Epizooties* 31 (2012): 199–210, www.oie.int/doc /ged/d11800.pdf; L. Guartdabassi, S. Schwarz, and D. H. Lloyd, "Pet Animals as Reservoirs of Antimicrobial-Resistant Bacteria," *Journal of Antimicrobial Chemotherapy* 54 (2004): 321–32, http://jac.oxfordjournals.org/content/54/2/321.full.pdf+html.

13. L. H. Kahn, B. Kaplan, and J. H. Steele, "Confronting Zoonoses through Closer Collaboration between Medicine and Veterinary Medicine (as `One Medicine')," *Veterinaria Italiana* 43 (2007): 5–19, www.te.izs.it/vet_italiana/2007/43_1/5_19.pdf.

14. Hippocrates, *On Airs, Waters, and Places*, http://classics.mit.edu/Hippocrates/airwatpl .html.

15. Ancient Asian health practitioners developed a procedure called "variolation" in which they took dried smallpox pus from lesions of people recovering from the disease and either scratched it into the skin or blew it into the nose of someone naive to smallpox (usually a young child). This practice reduced the mortality rate from 30 percent to 1–2 percent. But people still died from variolation. Dr. Jenner almost certainly got variolated as a child. He developed vaccination, a safer practice, by modifying variolation: he used dried cowpox pus instead of smallpox pus. U.S. National Library of Medicine, "Smallpox: A Great and Terrible Scourge," www.nlm.nih.gov/exhibition/smallpox/sp_variolation .html.

16. S. Riedel, "Edward Jenner and the History of Smallpox and Vaccination," *Baylor University Medical Center Proceedings* 18 (2005): 21–25, www.ncbi.nlm.nih.gov/pmc/articles/PMC 1200696/.

17. R. J. Dubos, *Louis Pasteur: Free Lance of Science* (Boston: Little, Brown, 1950), http:// archive.org/stream/louispasteurfree009068mbp#page/n7/mode/2up.

18. L. H. Kahn, "The End of Vaccines?" *Bulletin of the Atomic Scientists,* July 8, 2007, http://thebulletin.org/end-vaccines.

19. L. H. Kahn, "Confronting Zoonoses, Linking Human and Veterinary Medicine," *Emerging Infectious Diseases* 12 (2006): 556–61, http://wwwnc.cdc.gov/eid/article/12/4/05 -0956_article.htm.

20. National Research Council, *National Need and Priorities for Veterinarians in Biomedical Research* (Washington, DC: National Academies Press, 2004), www.nap.edu/openbook.php ?record_id=10878.

21. E. S. Anderson, "Drug Resistance in Salmonella typhimurium and Its Implications," *British Medical Journal* 3 (1968): 333–39; Joint Committee on the Use of Antibiotics in Animal Husbandry and Veterinary Medicine (The Swann Report), Cmnd. 4190. November 1969, Her Majesty's Stationery Office, London.

22. L. Backstrom, "Sweden's Ban on Antimicrobial Feed Additives Misunderstood," *Feedstuffs* 71, no. 48 (1999): 8; J. I. R. Castanon, "History of the Use of Antibiotic as Growth Promoters in European Poultry Feeds," *Poultry Science* 86 (2007): 2466–71.

23. Department of Health, Education and Welfare, Food and Drug Administration, 121 CFR Parf 1351, "Antibiotic and Sulfonamide Drugs in Animal Feeds," Proposed Statement of Policy, *Federal Register* 37, no. 21 (1972): 2444–45, http://google2.fda.gov/search

?q=cache:oJ6cWfcAFqcJ:www.fda.gov/ohrms/dockets/dailys/03/dec03/121203/03n-0324B
-sup0001-Tab-35-vol3.pdf+1972+Task+Force+Use+of+Antibiotics+in+Animal+Feeds&client
=FDAgov&site=FDAgov-OHRMS&lr=&proxystylesheet=FDAgov&output=xml_no_dtd&ie
=UTF-8&access=p&oe=UTF-8.

24. R. S. Lawrence, "The FDA Enters Withdrawal: The Future of Antibiotics on Farms,"
Atlantic, March 30, 2012, www.theatlantic.com/health/archive/2012/03/the-fda-enters
-withdrawal-the-future-of-antibiotics-on-farms/255236/.

25. White House, "National Strategy for Combating Antibiotic-Resistant Bacteria," www
.whitehouse.gov/sites/default/files/docs/carb_national_strategy.pdf.

26. WHO, World Health Day—7 April 2011, www.who.int/world-health-day/2011/en/;
N. Gilbert, "Rules Tighten on Use of Antibiotics on Farms," *Nature* 481, no. 7380 (2012): 125.

27. WHO, "Antimicrobial Resistance," Fact Sheet No. 194, updated April 2014, www.who
.int/mediacentre/factsheets/fs194/en/.

28. Editorial Board, "India and the Post-Antibiotic Era," *New York Times*, December 8, 2014,
www.nytimes.com/2014/12/09/opinion/india-and-the-post-antibiotic-era.html?src=twr.

29. UN Food and Agriculture Organization, "Feeding the Future," in *World Livestock
2011: Livestock in Food Security* (Rome, Italy: Author, 2011), pp. 78–80, www.fao.org/docrep
/014/i2373e/i2373e.pdf.

30. FAO Agriculture and Consumer Protection Dept. News, "FAO Symposium High-
lights the Importance of Enhancing Feed Conversion Efficiency for Ruminants," AAAP Animal Science Congress, November 26–30, 2012, Bangkok, www.fao.org/ag/againfo/home/en
/news_archive/2013_FAO_Symposium_highlights_importance_enhancing_feed_conversion
_efficiency.html.

31. P. J. Turnbaugh, R. E. Ley, M. Hamady, et al., "The Human Microbiome Project: Exploring the Microbial Part of Ourselves in a Changing World," *Nature* 449 (2007): 804–10,
www.ncbi.nlm.nih.gov/pmc/articles/PMC3709439/.

32. Institute of Medicine, *Antibiotic Resistance: Implications for Global Health and Novel
Intervention Strategies: Workshop Summary* (Washington DC: National Academies Press, 2010),
pp. 36–39, 4–5, www.nap.edu/catalog.php?record_id=12925.

33. Ibid., 41, 36–39.

34. Ibid., 2.

35. United Nations, Population Division of the Department of Economic and Social Affairs, "World Population to Reach 10 billion by 2100 if Fertility in All Countries Converges
to Replacement Level," 2010 Revision of World Population Prospects, May 3, 2011. There
are 58 high-fertility countries: Africa has 39, Asia has 9, Oceania has 6, and Latin America
has 4. High-variant projections place the world's population at 10.6 billion by 2050 and 15.8
billion by 2100. Low-variant projections estimate that the world's population will reach 8
billion by 2050 and decrease to 6 billion by 2100. http://esa.un.org/unpd/wpp/Documentation
/pdf/WPP2010_Press_Release.pdf.

36. S. DiGregorio, "Battle of the Dishes: Grass-Fed, Local Steak versus Supermarket
Steak," *Village Voice*, November 5, 2009, http://blogs.villagevoice.com/forkintheroad/2009
/11/battle_of_the_d_18.php.

37. F. M. Lappe, *Diet for a Small Planet* (New York: Ballantine Books, 1971); M. Pollan, *The
Omnivore's Dilemma: A Natural History of Four Meals* (New York: Penguin, 2006); M. Bittman,
Food Matters: A Guide to Conscious Eating with More Than 75 Recipes (New York: Simon & Schus-
ter, 2009); J. S. Foer, *Eating Animals* (Boston: Little, Brown, 2009); D. Barboza and S. Day, "Mc-
Donald's Seeking Cut in Antibiotics in Its Meat," *New York Times*, June 20, 2003, www.nytimes
.com/2003/06/20/business/mcdonald-s-seeking-cut-in-antibiotics-in-its-meat.html.

CHAPTER TWO: A Brief History of Meat Production and Antibiotics

1. W. J. Belasco, *Meals to Come: A History of the Future of Food* (Berkeley: University of California Press, 2006), pp. 4, 5; P. Singer, *Animal Liberation* (New York: HarperCollins, 1975); R. Southan, "The Enigma of Animal Suffering," *New York Times,* August 10, 2014, http://opinionator.blogs.nytimes.com/2014/08/10/how-similar-are-human-and-animal -suffering/?_php=true&_type=blogs&ref=opinion&_r=0.

2. F. Furuse, A. Suzuki, and H. Oshitani, "Origin of Measles Virus: Divergence from Rinderpest Virus between the 11th and 12th Centuries," *Virology Journal* 7 (2010), doi: 10.1186/1743-422X-7-52, www.virologyj.com/content/7/1/52; N. D. Wolfe, P. Daszak, A. M. Kilpatrick, and D. S. Burke, "Bushmeat Hunting, Deforestation, and Prediction of Zoonotic Disease," *Emerging Infectious Diseases* 11 (2005), doi:10.3201/eid1112.040789, http://wwwnc .cdc.gov/eid/article/11/12/04-0789_article.

3. V. Smil, "Meat in Human Evolution," chap. 2 in *Should We Eat Meat?: Evolution and Consequences of Modern Carnivory* (Chichester, UK: Wiley-Blackwell, 2013). See also R. Wrangham, *Catching Fire: How Cooking Made Us Human* (New York: Basic Books, 2009), pp. 116–20.

4. M. Ogle, *In Meat We Trust: An Unexpected History of Carnivore America* (New York: Houghton Mifflin Harcourt, 2013), chap. 1; M. Ogle, "Don't Like the American Way of Meat? Blame That First Thanksgiving Meal," *Time Magazine,* November 28, 2013, http:// ideas.time.com/2013/11/28/dont-like-the-american-way-of-meat-blame-that-first -thanksgiving-meal/.

5. Ogle, *In Meat We Trust,* 14–23, 30–40.

6. Ibid., 66–73.

7. T. G. Hall, "Wilson and the Food Crisis: Agricultural Price Control during World War I," *Agricultural History* 47, no. 1 (1973): 25–46.

8. A. Smith (Special Sanitary Commissioner), "The Stockyards and Packing Town; Insanitary Condition of the World's Largest Meat Market," *Lancet,* January 7, 1905, 49–52; A. Smith, "The Dark and Insanitary Premises Used for the Slaughtering of Cattle and Hogs— The Government Inspection," *Lancet,* January 14, 1905, 123; A. Smith, "Tuberculosis among the Stockyard Workers—Sanitation in Packingtown—The Police and the Dumping of Refuse—Vital Statistics," *Lancet,* January 21, 1905, 183–85; A. Smith, "Unhealthy Work in the Stockyards—Shameless Indifference to the Insanitary Condition of the Buildings and the Cattle Pens—For Legislative Interference," *Lancet,* January 28, 1905, 258–60. See also Ogle, *In Meat We Trust,* 74–81.

9. U. Sinclair, *The Jungle* (New York: Doubleday, 1906); editorial, "The Chicago Stockyards and the Meat Scandal," *Lancet,* June 9, 1906.

10. Hall, "Wilson and the Food Crisis"; J. H. Shideler, *Farm Crisis, 1919–1923* (Berkeley: University of California Press, 1957), pp. 10–19.

11. H.-J. Teuteberg, "Food Provisioning on the German Home Front, 1919–1918," in *Food and War in Twentieth Century Europe,* ed. I. Zweininger-Bargielowska, R. Duffett, and A. Drouard (Surrey, UK: Ashgate, 2011), pp. 59–71.

12. A. Offer, "The Blockade of Germany and the Strategy of Starvation, 1914–1918: An Agency Perspective," in *Great War, Total War: Combat and Mobilization on the Western Front, 1914–1918,* ed. Roger Chickering and Stig Forster (New York: Cambridge University Press, 2000), pp. 169–88.

13. Teuteberg, "Food Provisioning."

14. Hall, "Wilson and the Food Crisis."

15. Shideler, *Farm Crisis, 1919–1923,* pp. 10–19.

16. Hall, "Wilson and the Food Crisis."

17. Shideler, *Farm Crisis, 1919–1923*, p. 17; Ogle, *In Meat We Trust,* pp. 92–95; Alan L. Olmstead and Paul W. Rhode, "Beef, Veal, Pork, and Lamb—Slaughtering, Production, and Price: 1899–1999," in *Historical Statistics of the United States, Earliest Times to the Present: Millennial Edition,* ed. Susan B. Carter, Scott Sigmund Gartner, Michael R. Haines, Alan L. Olmstead, Richard Sutch, and Gavin Wright (New York: Cambridge University Press, 2006), table Da995-1019, http://hsus.cambridge.org/HSUSWeb/HSUSEntryServlet.

18. Shideler, *Farm Crisis, 1919–1923*, pp. 20–21, 37–40, 54.

19. R. Douglas Hurt, *American Agriculture: A Brief History* (West Lafayette, IN: Purdue University Press, 2002), 266–68.

20. Ibid.

21. Ibid., 287–330; Shideler, *Farm Crisis, 1919–1923*, pp. 282–83; U.S. Bureau of the Census, table 1, Urban and Rural Population: 1900 to 1990, released 1995, https://www.census .gov/population/censusdata/urpop0090.txt (accessed September 10, 2014).

22. Shideler, *Farm Crisis 1919–1923*, pp. 282–83; Olmstead and Rhode, "Beef, Veal, Pork, and Lamb."

23. Hurt, *American Agriculture*, p. 291.

24. Ibid., pp. 294, 320–21, 362.

25. C. D. Berdanier, "Food Shortages during World War II: Can We Learn from This Experience?" *Nutrition Today,* 41 (2006): 160–63.

26. L. Collingham, *The Taste of War: World War Two and the Battle for Food* (London: Penguin Books, 2011), pp. 431–32.

27. Olmstead and Rhode, "Beef, Veal, Pork, and Lamb"; Alan L. Olmstead and Paul W. Rhode, "Chickens, Turkeys, and Eggs—Number, Production, Price, Sales, and Value per Head: 1909–1999 [Annual]," in Carter et al., *Historical Statistics of the United States,* table Da1039-1058; Ogle, *In Meat We Trust,* pp. 108–9.

28. Ogle, *In Meat We Trust,* pp. 108–9.

29. T. H. Carpenter, "Biographical Article: Thomas Hughes Jukes (1906–1999)," *Journal of Nutrition* 130 (2000): 1521–23; T. H. Jukes, "Public Health Significance of Feeding Low Levels of Antibiotics to Animals," *Advances in Applied Microbiology* 16 (1973): 1–30.

30. Jukes, "Public Health Significance," 3.

31. Ibid.

32. I. Trehan, H. S. Goldbach, L. N. LaGrone, et al., "Antibiotics as Part of the Management of Severe Acute Malnutrition," *New England Journal of Medicine* 368 (2013): 425–35, www.nejm.org/doi/full/10.1056/NEJMoa1202851; I. N. Okeke, J. R. Cruz, and G. T. Keusch, "Antibiotics for Uncomplicated Severe Malnutrition," letters to the editor, *New England Journal of Medicine* 368 (2013): 2435–37, www.nejm.org/doi/full/10.1056/NEJMoa1202851#t =letters. See also A. Bowen and R. V. Tauxe, "Antibiotics for Uncomplicated Severe Malnutrition," letters to the editor, *New England Journal of Medicine* 368 (2013): 2435–37, www.nejm .org/doi/full/10.1056/NEJMoa1202851#t=letters.

33. Olmstead and Rhode, "Chickens, Turkeys, and Eggs"; A. S. Blinder, "The Anatomy of Double-Digit Inflation in the 1970's," in *Inflation: Causes and Effects,* ed. R. E. Hall (Chicago: University of Chicago Press, 1982), pp. 261–82, www.nber.org/chapters/c11462.pdf.

34. USDA Economic Research Service, Food Expenditures, table 7, Column H, www.ers .usda.gov/data-products/food-expenditures.aspx#.VAnM6P2jShM; FAO Statistics, Food Security Indicators, Access, Share of food expenditure of the poor, V 2.7, www.fao.org/economic /ess/ess-fs/ess-fadata/en/#.VRFgGjTF9nh.

35. T. Watanabe, "Infective Heredity of Multiple Drug Resistance in Bacteria," *Bacteriological Reviews* 27, no. 1 (1963): 87–115.

CHAPTER THREE: The British Experience

1. J. Pearce, "E. S. Anderson Dies at 94; Cautioned on Antibiotics," *New York Times,* April 1, 2006, www.nytimes.com/2006/04/01/world/europe/01anderson.html?fta=y.

2. Bacteriophages were used in the 1960s to identify bacteria. A specific strain of *Salmonella typhimurium* was identified by a single phage, type 29, and was referred to by this nomenclature: *S. typhimurium* type 29. This organism does not cause disease as severe for humans as does *Salmonella typhi.*

3. E. S. Anderson, "Drug Resistance in Salmonella typhimurium and Its Implications," *British Medical Journal* 3 (1968): 333–39.

4. Ibid.

5. Ibid.

6. Ibid.

7. V. P. Geoghegan, "A Milk-borne Outbreak of Food Poisoning Due to Salmonella typhimurium," *Medical Officer* 114 (1965): 73–74.

8. Anderson, "Drug Resistance in Salmonella typhimurium," 339. In a postscript, Dr. Anderson noted, "This could be done if a different range of antibiotics were used in animals from those used in man, and if the two groups of antibiotics gave no cross-resistance to each other. The occurrence of enterobacteria in man which showed resistance to antibiotics of the animal range would then indicate that the resistance had originated in animals."

9. James Turner (1908–1980), First Baron of Netherthorpe and president of the National Farmer's Union (1945–1960), chaired a joint committee established in 1960 by the Agricultural and Medical Research Councils, which examined the potential dangers of feeding antibiotics to farm animals. In 1962 the committee published its first report, stating that the only potential hazard to human and animal health would be the effects of antibiotics on bacterial populations. It recommended that the Therapeutic Substances Act (Supply of Antibiotics for Agricultural Purposes) of 1953 be continued and extended to include young calves. These regulations stipulated that prescriptions should not be needed for feed containing antibiotics. See also R. Braude, "Antibiotics in Animal Feeds in Great Britain," *Journal of Animal Science* 46 (1978): 1425–36, www.animal-science.org/content/46/5/1425.short.

10. Joint Committee on the Use of Antibiotics in Animal Husbandry and Veterinary Medicine (the Swann Report), Cmnd. 4190, November 1969, Her Majesty's Stationery Office, London, p. 6. See also P. W. Daykin, "Antibiotic Usage in Veterinary Practice before Swann," in *Ten Years on from Swann* (papers given at a symposium organized by the Association of Veterinarians in Industry, October 5–6, 1981), ed. D. W. Jolly, D. J. S. Miller, D. B. Ross, et al. (Surrey, UK: Gresham Press, 1981), pp. 27–35.

11. M. H. Fussell, "Antibiotics as Growth Promoters," in *Ten Years on from Swann,* pp. 43–49.

12. J. S. Kiser, "A Perspective on the Use of Antibiotics in Animal Feeds," *Journal of Animal Science* 42 (1976): 1058–72, www.animal-science.org/content/42/4/1058.abstract.

13. Joint Committee, Swann Report, chap. 1, p. 11.

14. Kiser, "Use of Antibiotics."

15. Joint Committee, Swann Report, chap. 12, "Summary and Recommendations"; Medicines Act 1968, chap. 67. (The committee that the Swann Report referred to was the Medicines Commission established by the Medicines Act of 1968 [National Archives, www.legislation.gov.uk/ukpga/1968/67/enacted]). Note: One year before the Swann Report was published, Parliament passed the Medicines Act of 1968, which established a Medicines Commission, appointed by the ministers of Health and Agriculture, to oversee the licensing

and practice of medicine, veterinary medicine, and pharmacy and to advise the ministers regarding the execution of the legislation. The act included the oversight of clinical trials and medicinal tests on animals and the use of "medicated animal feeding stuffs," but it did not limit the use of antibiotics in livestock.

16. L.-E. Edqvist and K. P. Pedersen, "Antimicrobials as Growth Promoters: Resistance to Common Sense," in *Late Lessons from Early Warnings: The Precautionary Principle, 1896–2000,* ed. P. Harremoes, D. Gee, M. MacGarvin, et al. (Copenhagen: European Environmental Agency, 2001), Issue Report 22, chap. 9, www.eea.europa.eu/publications/environmental _issue_report_2001_22.

17. Kiser, "Use of Antibiotics."

18. R. Young, A. Cowe, C. Nunan, J. Harvey, and L. Mason, "The Use and Misuse of Antibiotics in UK Agriculture, Part 2: Antibiotic Resistance and Human Health," Soil Association, Bristol, UK, 1999, www.soilassociation.org/LinkClick.aspx?fileticket=RcHBJXC1Mxc%3D &tabid=1715.

19. British House of Commons, "Use of Antibiotics in Animal Husbandry and Veterinary Medicine (Swann Report)," HC Debate, November 20, 1969, vol. 791 cc1525-31, http://hansard.millbanksystems.com/commons/1969/nov/20/use-of-antibiotics-in-animal -husbandry.

20. L. Amey, "Three Antibiotics Banned from Animal Food," *London Times,* November 21, 1969.

21. J. Howie, "The Situation in the U.K.—Then and Now," in *Ten Years on from Swann,* pp. 3–7.

22. Braude, "Antibiotics in Animal Feeds."

23. Editorial, "Death of a Quango," *British Medical Journal* 282 (1981): 1413–14.

24. E. J. Threlfall, L. R. Ward, and B. Row, "Spread of Multiresistant Strains of Salmonella typhimurium phage Types 204 and 193 in Britain," *British Medical Journal* 2, no. 6143 (1978): 997; Editorial, "Why Has Swann Failed?" *British Medical Journal* 280, no. 6225 (1980): 1195–96.

25. Howie, "Situation in the U.K."

26. E. John Threlfall, former director of the Laboratory of Enteric Pathogens, Centre for Infections, UK Health Protection Agency, personal communication, July 3, 2012.

27. Veterinary Medicines Directorate, Department for the Environment, Food, and Rural Affairs, Publications, "Sales of Antimicrobial Products Authorised for Use as Veterinary Medicines, Antiprotozoals, Antifungals and Coccidiostats in the UK," www.noah.co.uk /papers/antimicrosales1998.htm. Sales data from 1993 to 1997 includes products used in a combination of food and nonfood items. Changes in the analysis methodology after 1997 prohibit comparisons with sales data for subsequent years.

28. Veterinary Medicines Directorate, "Sales of Antimicrobial Products Authorized for Use as Veterinary Medicines in the UK," 2003 Report, p. 13; 2006 Report, p. 14; "UK Veterinary Antibiotic Resistance and Sales Surveillance," 2013 Report, p. 30, https://www.gov.uk /government/uploads/system/uploads/attachment_data/file/382991/VARSS.pdf.

29. From 1993 to 2004, data was voluntarily provided by veterinary pharmaceutical companies marketing antibiotics in the United Kingdom. In 2005 Veterinary Medicine Regulations required veterinary pharmaceutical companies to provide sales data for products for which they had marketing authorizations. Data collected by the Veterinary Medicines Directorate, "Sales of Antimicrobial Products Authorised for Use as Veterinary Medicines, Antiprotozoals, Antifungals and Coccidiostats in the UK" and personal communication with the Antimicrobial Resistance Team, Veterinary Medicines Directorate, DEFRA, UK, August 3, 2012; Veterinary Medicines Directorate, "UK Veterinary Antibiotic Resistance and

Sales Surveillance," 2013 Report, p. 30, https://www.gov.uk/government/uploads/system/uploads/attachment_data/file/382991/VARSS.pdf.

30. Veterinary Medicines Directorate, "Sales of Antimicrobial Products Authorized for Use as Veterinary Medicines in the UK," 2011 Report, p. 28.

31. Merck Veterinary Manual, "Overview of Coccidiosis in Poultry," www.merckvetmanual.com/mvm/poultry/coccidiosis/overview_of_coccidiosis_in_poultry.html. Coccidia parasites are ubiquitous in poultry production, causing birds to become sick after ingesting oocysts from the droppings of infected or recovered birds. Oocysts are thick-walled structures in which parasite zygotes develop; they infect various sites in birds' intestines. These oocysts contaminate soil, water, feed, equipment, clothing, farm workers, and other animals. They are killed by high temperatures or freezing but are resistant to some disinfectants. Sick birds develop severe diarrhea, weight loss, and decreased egg production. Mortality rates are high. Coccidiostats are drugs used to prevent infection and economic loss.

Necrotic enteritis is a deadly intestinal infection caused by the toxin-producing bacteria *Clostridium perfringens*.

32. Veterinary Medicines Directorate, "Sales of Antimicrobial Products Authorized for Use as Veterinary Medicines in the UK," 2003 Report, p. 16; 2006 Report, p. 17; "UK Veterinary Antibiotic Resistance and Sales Surveillance," 2013 Report, p. 22, https://www.gov.uk/government/uploads/system/uploads/attachment_data/file/382991/VARSS.pdf.

33. Veterinary Medicines Directorate, "Sales of Antimicrobial Products Authorized for Use as Veterinary Medicines in the UK," 2003 Report, p. 24; 2006 Report, p. 24; "UK Veterinary Antibiotic Resistance and Sales Surveillance," 2013 Report, pp. 26, 31, http://webarchive.nationalarchives.gov.uk/20140909112428/, www.vmd.defra.gov.uk/pharm/antibiotic_sales data.aspx, https://www.gov.uk/government/uploads/system/uploads/attachment_data/file/382991/VARSS.pdf.

34. E. J. Threlfall, "Epidemic Salmonella typhimurium DT 104—a Truly International Multiresistant Clone," *Journal of Antimicrobial Chemotherapy* 46 (2000): 7–10; S. Evans and R. Davies, "Case Control Study of Multiple-Resistant *Salmonella typhimurium* DT 104 Infection of Cattle in Great Britain," *Veterinary Record* 238 (1996): 557–58.

35. A. E. Mather, L. Matthews, D. J. Mellor, et al., "An Ecological Approach to Assessing the Epidemiology of Antimicrobial Resistance in Animal and Human Populations," *Proceedings of the Royal Society of London B* 279 (2012): 1630–39, http://rspb.royalsocietypublishing.org/content/early/2011/11/10/rspb.2011.1975, published November 16, 2011, online, doi: 10.1098/rspb.2011.1975.

36. P. Collignon, "Antibiotic Resistance in Human *Salmonella* Isolates Are Related to Animal Strains," *Proceedings of the Royal Society of London B* 279 (2012): 2922–23, http://rspb.royalsocietypublishing.org/content/279/1740/2922.

37. A. E. Mather, L. Matthews, D. J. Mellor, et al., "The Diversity of Antimicrobial Resistance Is Different in Salmonella Typhimurium DT 104 from Co-located Animals and Humans," *Proceedings of the Royal Society of London B* 279 (2012): 2924–25.

38. British Veterinary Association, "New Research Suggests Animals Not to Blame for Human Antimicrobial Resistance," www.beva.org.uk/news-and-events/news/view/185.

39. J. Laurance, "Death Wish: Routine Use of Vital Antibiotics on Farms Threatens Human Health," *Independent*, June 17, 2011, www.independent.co.uk/life-style/health-and-families/health-news/death-wish-routine-use-of-vital-antibiotics-on-farms-threatens-human-health-2298761.html#.

40. National Office of Animal Health, "Antibiotic Resistance," www.noah.co.uk/issues/briefingdoc/11-abres.htm.

41. K. Hoelzer, A. Switt, and M. Wiedmann, "Animal Contact as a Source of Human Non-typhoidal Salmonellosis," *Veterinary Research* 42 (2011): 34, www.veterinaryresearch .org/content/42/1/34; K. S. Harker, C. Lane, E. De Pinna, et al., "An Outbreak of *Salmonella typhiumurium* DT 191a Associated with Reptile Feeder Mice," *Epidemiology Infections* 139 (2011): 1254–61.

CHAPTER FOUR: Lessons from Sweden

1. The specific antibiotics used as feed additives included avoparcin, bacitracin, nitrovin, oleandromycin, and spiramycin. Quinoxalines and streptogramins were given separately. SVARM 2000, National Veterinary Institute, Uppsala, Sweden, www.sva.se/globalassets/rede sign2011/pdf/om_sva/publikationer/trycksaker/1/svarm2000.pdf, p. 14, table AC V, notes 1, 4; L. Backstrom, "Sweden's Ban on Antimicrobial Feed Additives Misunderstood," *Feedstuffs* 71, no. 48 (1999): 8; R. Carson, *Silent Spring* (New York: Houghton Mifflin, 1962). Rachel Carson's best-selling book raised global awareness about the deleterious impact of pesticides on the environment. See also E. Griswold, "How `Silent Spring' Ignited the Environmental Movement," *New York Times*, September 21, 2012, www.nytimes.com/2012/09/23/magazine/how -silent-spring-ignited-the-environmental-movement.html?ref=business.

2. Backstrom, "Sweden's Ban Misunderstood."

3. T. Michelsen, "Ar Griskottet Farlight Att Ata? 30 ton antibiotika till de svenska slaktdjuren varje ar" (Pork is safe to eat? 30 tons of antibiotics to the Swedish slaughter animals each year), *Dagens Nyheter,* November 1, 1981.

4. Gunnela Stahle, agronomist, Economic Policy Division, Federation of Swedish Farmers, telephone conversation, March 19, 2013.

5. Ibid.

6. The Feedingstuffs Act (1985:295) went into effect in 1986.

7. J. Inborr, "Swedish Poultry Production without In-Feed Antibiotics—A Testing Ground or a Model for the Future?" Proceedings, Australian Poultry Science Symposium, Sydney, Australia, 2000, pp. 1–9, www.vetsci.usyd.edu.au/apss/documents/2000/APSS2000 -inborr-pp1-9.pdf.

8. Ibid; Stahle, telephone conversation, March 19, 2013.

9. Gunnela Stahle, "The Swedish Model of Animal Production: Economic Effects on Swedish Farming," Lantbrukarnas Riksforbund (Federation of Swedish farmers), August 28, 1998, presented at Swedish Ministry of Agriculture, Food and Fisheries Seminar, Stockholm, Sweden, September 3–4, 1998.

10. SVARM 2004, p. 11, table AC III.

11. Swedish Antibiotic Utilization and Resistance in Human Medicine and Swedish Veterinary Antimicrobial Resistance Monitoring (SWEDRES)/SVARM 2013, Public Health Agency of Sweden, Solna Sweden, and Swedish National Veterinary Institute, Uppsala, Sweden. ISSN 1650-6332, p. 40, table 1.9, www.sva.se/en/Antibiotika/SVARM-reports/.

12. Stahle, telephone conversation, March 19, 2013.

13. M. Wierup, "The Swedish Experience of the 1986 Year Ban of Antimicrobial Growth Promoters, with Special Reference to Animal Health, Disease Prevention, Productivity, and Usage of Antimicrobials," *Microbial Drug Resistance* 7 (2001): 183–190, www.ncbi.nlm.nih .gov/pubmed/11442345; see also J. Bates, Z. Jordens, and J. B. Selkon, "Evidence for an Animal Origin of Vancomycin-Resistant Enterococci," *Lancet* 342 (1993): 490–91; H. W. Smith and J. E. Tucker, "The Effect of Antimicrobial Feed Additives on the Colonization of the Alimentary Tract of Chickens by Salmonella typhimurium," *Journal of Hygiene* 80 (1978): 217–31, www.ncbi.nlm.nih.gov/pmc/articles/PMC2129995/.

14. National Veterinary Institute, "Swedish Veterinary Antimicrobial Resistance Monitoring 2000," p. 13, www.sva.se/upload/Redesign2011/Pdf/Om_SVA/publikationer/Trycksaker/1/svarm2000.pdf; *Salmonella* control in Sweden (Svensk Fågel), www.svenskfagel.se/?p=2216.

15. Christina Greko, DVM, PhD, associate professor, Department of Animal Health and Antimicrobial Strategies, National Veterinary Institute, Sweden, personal communication, March 12, 2012. Sweden has been aggressive with *Salmonella* control. Beginning in 1941, the country started a voluntary program to control fowl typhoid (*Salmonella gallinarium/pullorum*). A severe salmonella epidemic in 1953 to 1954 prompted a government regulation in 1961 mandating stricter *Salmonella* control with the objective that all animal products meant for human consumption would be free of *Salmonella*. Salmonella is a reportable disease; all veterinary laboratories are required to immediately report any *Salmonella* isolates to the Swedish Board of Agriculture; the isolates are sent to the National Veterinary Institute for testing. A *Salmonella* control program targeting poultry began in 1970 after a series of severe human outbreaks originating in chickens. Since 1984–85, producers receive compensation from insurance companies if their flocks must be destroyed after testing positive for *Salmonella*. In addition to the control of *Salmonella* in livestock, there is also a program for factories that produce feed for farm animals. All animal feed must be free of *Salmonella;* samples are sent to the National Veterinary Institute for testing. *Salmonella* Control Program in Sweden (Svensk fagel), www.svenskfagel.se/?p=2216. See also B. George, C. L. Quarles, and D. L. Fagerberg, "Virginiamycin Effects on Controlling Necrotic Enteritis Infection in Chickens," *Poultry Science* 61 (1982): 447–450, www.ncbi.nlm.nih.gov/pubmed/6806795.

16. In 1993 *Lancet* published a letter to the editor reporting evidence linking the use of avoparcin in livestock, particularly poultry, with the emergence of vancomycin-resistant enterococci in humans. The authors found VRE ubiquitous in raw sewage, poultry and pigs, and fresh and frozen chickens. This and subsequent studies were published after Sweden had already stopped using avoparcin. Bates, Jordens, and Selkon, "Evidence for an Animal Origin."

17. L. R. McDougald and S. H. Fitz-Coy, "Coccidiosis," in *Diseases of Poultry,* 13th ed., ed. D. E. Swayne (Oxford: Wiley-Blackwell, 2013), pp. 1148–49. Tissue damage from coccidiosis infections increases the risk of enteral colonization by *C. perfringens,* leading to necrotic enteritis. Almost all young poultry are given continuous medications with low levels of anticoccidial drugs to prevent these diseases. In the United States, sales of preventive medications exceed $90 million; more than $300 million is spent worldwide.

18. Greko, personal communication, March 12, 2012. Coccidiostats are ionophores, a class of antibiotics that has never been used in humans.

19. SWEDRES/SVARM 2012, p. 39, table 5.10, www.sva.se/globalassets/redesign2011/pdf/om_sva/publikationer/swedres_svarm2012.pdf. Data for 2012 was not available during the analysis of this book.

20. Stahle, telephone conversation, March 19, 2013. See Wierup, "Swedish Experience of 1986 Ban."

21. Wierup, "Swedish Experience of 1986 Ban."

22. J. W. Smith, M. D. Tokach, R. D. Goodband, et al., "The Effects of Increasing Zinc Oxide on Growth Performance of Weanling Pigs," *Professional Animal Scientist* 14 (1998), pp. 197–200, http://pas.fass.org/content/14/4/197.full.pdf+html.

23. Ibid. See also Ministry of Enterprise and Innovation, Swedish Government Official Report, *Antimicrobial Feed Additives,* chap. 2, "Background," 1997, p. 27, www.government.se/sb/d/574/a/54899.

24. SVARM reports after 2008 inexplicably did not include zinc oxide sales. The data was either not collected or not made public. C. Jondreville, P. S. Revy, and J. Y. Dourmad,

"Dietary Means to Better Control the Environmental Impact of Copper and Zinc by Pigs from Weaning to Slaughter," *Liverstock Production Science* 84 (2003): 147–56.

25. Stahle, "Swedish Model of Animal Production: Economic Effects on Swedish Farming." The study compared production costs between the most competent Swedish and Danish farmers. As a result of the new regulations (antibiotic ban and animal welfare requirements), production costs would be slightly more than 1 SEK (Swedish kroner) per kilogram of pig meat (approximately 15 cents in 1998 USD according to Trading Economics, www.tradingeconomics.com/sweden/currency), higher in Sweden than in Denmark, not accounting for differences in taxes, fees, and other costs. Most of the cost differences were in weaner (young pig) production.

26. Data obtained from Asa Lannhard Oberg, market analyst, Department of Trade and Markets, Swedish Board of Agriculture, personal communication, September 5, 2013.

27. Ibid., September 4, October 16, 2013.

28. Jimmie Enhall, Statistics Unit, Swedish Board of Agriculture, personal communication, June 25, 2013.

29. Oberg, personal communication, October 16, 2013.

30. Enhall, personal communication, June 25, June 18, 2013.

31. Cattle farms, particularly dairy cattle farms, decreased as well. From 1980 to 2012, cattle farms decreased by 70 percent and dairy cattle farms by 89 percent. SWEDRES/SVARM 2012, p. 91, table 7.7.

32. Statistics Sweden 2012, Swedish Board of Agriculture, Swedish Environmental Protection Agency, and Federation of Swedish Farmers, *Sustainability in Swedish Agriculture 2012,* p. 16, fig. 7, www.scb.se/statistik/_publikationer/MI1305_2012A01_BR_MI72BR1201.pdf. Cattle farming decreased as well.

33. SWEDRES/SVARM 2012, pp. 91–92, tables 7.6, 7.7, and 7.8.

34. Statistics Sweden 2012, *Sustainability in Swedish Agriculture 2012,* p. 17, fig. 10. Neither pork production after the mid-1980s nor beef production after 1990 could meet consumer demand.

35. Stahle, e-mail correspondence, July 26, 2013.

36. Swedish National Veterinary Institute, Swedish Veterinary Antimicrobial Resistance Monitoring System, www.sva.se/en/Antibiotika/SVARM-reports/; and Swedish Institute for Communicable Disease Control, Report on Swedish Antibiotic Utilization and Resistance in Human Medicine, www.smittskyddsinstitutet.se/publikationer/arsrapporter -och-verksamhetsberattelser/swedres/.

37. Swedish National Veterinary Institute, Swedish Veterinary Antimicrobial Resistance Monitoring System, www.sva.se/en/Antibiotika/SVARM-reports/; SVARM 2000, pp. 4–6. *Enterococcus* (*Enterococcus faecium* and *Enterococcus faecalis*) bacteria are discussed in depth in chapter 5.

38. Surveillance and antibiotic susceptibility testing methodologies and classifications are described in detail in each SVARM and SWEDRES report available on the Internet.

39. SVARM 2011, p. 17, table SALM V. Note: In SVARM 2002, p. 15, table S III, the resistance rate against streptomycin was reported as 78 percent and against tetracycline as 14 percent. The more recently reported numbers are used in this book.

40. SVARM 2011, p. 54. Salmonella in animals is a notifiable disease in Sweden. The SVARM data comes from isolates submitted for mandatory antibiotic susceptibility testing. Also, some isolates are collected at slaughter (neck skins, carcass swabs, etc.) as part of the *Salmonella* surveillance program.

41. SWEDRES/SVARM 2012, p. 56. For the *S. typhimurium* isolates collected from farm animals from 2000 to 2012, 39 percent were from pigs, 32 percent from cattle, 27 percent

from poultry, and 2 percent from sheep. Relatively few (10 percent) were multiresistant to antibiotics; the majority (74 percent) were susceptible to all antibiotics tested.

42. SVARM 2000, p. 14, table AC V. Note: Antibiotics used as growth-promoting agents included nitroimidazoles (QP51AA), quinoxalines, streptogramins (e.g., virginiamycin), avoparcin, bacitracin, nitrovin, oleandromycin, and spiramycin. Streptomycin is an aminoglycoside. Other aminoglycosides include gentamicin, neomycin, and apramycin. See also Ministry of Enterprise and Innovation, Swedish Government Official Report, *Antimicrobial Feed Additives*, chap. 2, "Background," 1997, pp. 30–31.

43. SWEDRES/SVARM 2012, p. 58, table 6.12.

44. K. Eld, A. Gunnarsson, T. Holmberg, et al., "Salmonella Isolated from Animals and Feedstuffs in Sweden during 1983–1987," *Acta Veterinaria Scandinavica* 32 (1991): 261–77.

45. SWEDRES/SVARM 2012, pp. 22 and 38.

46. Ibid., pp. 22,58–59, tables 6.12 and 6.14; SWEDRES reports: 2002, p. 20; 2003, p. 22; 2004, p. 23; 2005, p. 25; 2006, p. 27; 2007, p. 28; 2008, p. 28; SVARM 2011, p. 17, table SALM V.

47. According to Statistics Sweden, Sweden's population in 2012 was 9.56 million. www .scb.se/en_/Finding-statistics/Statistics-by-subject-area/Population/Population-composition /Population-statistics/Aktuell-Pong/25795/Yearly-statistics--The-whole-country/26040/. The total number of livestock in Sweden in 2012 (cattle, sheep, pigs, and laying hens) was 11.76 million, according to the 2012 SWEDRES/SVARM report, p. 91.

48. SWEDRES/SVARM 2012, p. 12.

49. Ibid., p. 19.

50. Ibid., pp. 38–39, tables 5.8, 5.9, and 5.10.

51. Ibid., p. 39, table 5.10.

CHAPTER FIVE: Lessons from Denmark

1. B. E. Murray, "Editorial Response: What Can We Do about Vancomycin-Resistant Enterococci?" *Clinical Infectious Diseases* 20 (1995): 1134–36; R. Leclercq, E. Derlot, J. Duval, et al., "Plasmid-mediated Resistance to Vancomycin and Teicoplanin in Enterococcus Faecium," *New England Journal of Medicine* 319 (1988): 157–61. See also A. H. Uttley, C. H. Collins, J. Naidoo, et al., "Vancomycin-Resistant Enterococci," *Lancet* 331 (1988): 57–58.

2. Ampicillin-resistant enterococci preceded VRE by many years. Enterococci are Gram-positive bacteria that normally reside in the intestines of humans and animals and in the environment. Both *E. faecium* and *Enterococcus faecalis* are common in the human gut. In livestock, *E. faecium* predominates. These bacteria can cause urinary tract infections, endocarditis, surgical wound infections, bacteremia, and neonatal sepsis. Antibiotic resistance in these bacteria is well documented. See K. Fisher and C. Phillips, "The Ecology, Epidemiology and Virulence of Enterococcus," *Microbiology* 155 (2009): 1749–57, http://mic.sgmjournals .org/content/155/6/1749.full.pdf+html. Reports in both *Lancet* and the *New England Journal of Medicine* involved seriously ill patients with acute leukemia and end-stage renal failure, respectively. The French patients with acute leukemia had not been treated with vancomycin but had undergone digestive tract decontamination involving multiple antibiotics in preparation for bone marrow transplants. Two strains of VRE were isolated from the leukemia patients' feces, and their resistance genes were located in structurally related plasmids. In London, 22 patients with end-stage renal failure or multiple organ failure with acute renal failure had VRE isolated from blood and/or body fluids. Fifty-five strains of VRE were identified, and many of them were resistant to multiple antibiotics.

3. Leclercq et al., "Plasmid-mediated Resistance"; Uttley et al., "Vancomycin-Resistant Enterococci"; M. B. Edmond, J. F. Ober, D. L. Weinbaum, et al., "Vancomycin-Resistant *En-*

terococcus faecium Bacteremia: Risk Factors for Infection," *Clinical Infectious Diseases* 20 (1995): 1126–33, http://cid.oxfordjournals.org/content/20/5/1126.short. See also Murray, "Editorial Response."

4. J. Bates, J. Z. Jordens, and D. T. Griffiths, "Farm Animals as a Putative Reservoir for Vancomycin-Resistant Enterococcal Infection in Man," *Journal of Antimicrobial Chemotherapy* 34 (1994): 507–16; I. Klare, H. Heier, H. Claus, et al., "VanA-mediated High-level Glycopeptide Resistance in Enterococcus faecium from Animal Husbandry," *FEMS Microbiology Letters* 125 (1995): 165–72, http://onlinelibrary.wiley.com/doi/10.1111/j.1574-6968.1995.tb07353.x /abstract.

5. Klare et al., "VanA-mediated Glycopeptide Resistance"; F. M. Aarestrup, "Occurrence, Selection and Spread of Resistance to Antimicrobial Agents Used for Growth Promotion for Food Animals in Denmark," *APMIS,* Suppl. 101, 108 (2000): 5–6.

6. I. Klare, H. Heier, H. Claus, et al., "Enterococcus faecium Strains with vanA-mediated High-level Glycopeptide Resistance Isolated from Animal Foodstuffs and Fecal Samples of Humans in the Community," *Microbial Drug Resistance* 1 (1995): 265–72, http://online .liebertpub.com/doi/abs/10.1089/mdr.1995.1.265.

7. Erythromycin has a spectrum of activity similar to that of penicillin. It is used when individuals are allergic to penicillin. *Enterococci* have developed resistance to erythromycin as well as to penicillin. A. Portillo, F. Ruiz-Larrea, et al., "Macrolide Resistance Genes in Enterococcus spp. Antimicrobial Agents," *Chemotherapy* 44 (April 2000): 967–71.

8. Danish Integrated Antimicrobial Resistance Monitoring and Research Program (DANMAP) 2012, p. 95, www.danmap.org/Downloads/Reports.aspx.

9. FDA drug safety information, www.fda.gov/Drugs/DrugSafety/PostmarketDrugSafety InformationforPatientsandProviders/ucm101503.htm. See also D. R. Allington and M. P. Rivey, "Quinupristin/dalfopristin: A Therapeutic Review," *Clinical Therapeutics* 23 (January 2001): 24–44.

10. F. Aarestrup, "Get Pigs off Antibiotics," *Nature* 486 (2012): 465–66.

11. Frank Aarestrup, professor of microbiology and head of the EU Reference Laboratory for Antimicrobial Resistance, and the WHO Collaborating Centre for Antimicrobial Resistance in Foodborne Pathogens at the National Food Institute, Technical University of Denmark, Lyngby, Denmark, e-mail correspondence, November 5, 2013.

12. Aarestrup, "Occurrence, Selection and Spread of Resistance.".

13. Teleconference with Nicolaj Norgaard, director; Martin Andersson, head of department, board secretary; and Niels Jorgen Kjeldsen, head of department, Nutrition and Reproduction, Pig Research Centre, Danish Agriculture and Food Council, November 6, 2013.

14. Aarestrup, "Occurrence, Selection and Spread."

15. DANMAP No. 1, February 1997, p. 3. Details on how the data is collected and analyzed are available in each DANMAP report.

16. F. M. Aarestrup, "Consumption of Antimicrobial Growth Promoters," *APMIS,* Suppl. 101, 108 (2000): 8, table 2.

17. H. C. Wegener, "Letter: Historical Yearly Usage of Glycopeptides for Animals and Humans: The American-European Paradox Revisited," *Antimicrobial Agents and Chemotherapy* 42 (1998): 3049; Aarestrup, "Consumption of Antimicrobial Growth Promoters," 8, table 3.

18. The greatest volume of growth promoters in feedstuffs was used in finisher pigs. In 1997 the principal antibiotic growth-promoter agent in finisher pigs was 20 mg/kg tylosin (maximum). Tylosin is a macrolide, similar to erythromycin. On average, feedstuffs contained approximately 22 mg of active ingredients. WHO International Review Panel's Evaluation of the Termination of the Use of Antimicrobial Growth Promoters in Denmark,

"Impacts of Antimicrobial Growth Promoter Termination in Denmark," Foulum, Denmark. November 2002, p. 18, note, www.who.int/gfn/links/gssamrgrowthreportstory/en/.

19. Streptogramin antibiotics include virginiamycin, pristinamycin, and quinupristin/dalfopristin. They inhibit bacterial protein synthesis. www.ncbi.nlm.nih.gov/pubmed/10197038.

20. WHO International Review Panel, "Impacts of Growth Promoter Termination," pp. 9, 10. The pig industry continued to use zinc oxide to prevent diarrhea. Farmers were required to obtain a veterinarian's prescription for a typical dose of 2,000 to 5,000 parts per million, up to 14 days after weaning. Unfortunately, there is no surveillance data on the use of zinc oxide in pigs. The only data available, according to Jorgen Schlundt, director of the Danish National Food Institute, is from the Danish environmental agency's 2001 estimate that approximately 1,200 tons of zinc were spread through slurry from pigs.

21. WHO International Review Panel, "Impacts of Growth Promoter Termination."

22. Ibid., p. 6.

23. Ibid., pp. 6–7; DANMAP 2000, p. 11, table 4; 2010, p. 30, table 4.2; 2012, p. 29, table 4.1; 2009, p. 25, table 5; 2010, p. 30, table 4.2; 2012, p. 29, table 4.1.

24. DANMAP 2010, p. 28.

25. DANMAP 2009, p. 25, table 5; 2010, p. 30, table 4.2; 2012, p. 25, table 4.1; 2013, p. 26, table 4.1.

26. DANMAP 2012, p. 26.

27. G. Gyton, "Denmark Plans to Halve Antibiotic Use in Pigs," *Global Meat News,* October 28, 2014, www.globalmeatnews.com/Industry-Markets/Denmark-plans-to-halve-tetracycline-antibiotic-use-in-pigs.

28. DANMAP 2002, pp. 21–24; 2005, p. 43; 2006, p. 40; 2012, p. 63, table 6.2; 2013, p. 56, table 6.2.

29. I. A. Onwuezobe, P. O. Oshun, and C. C. Odigwe, "Antimicrobials for Treating Symptomatic Non-typhoidal Salmonella Infection," *Cochrane Database Systematic Reviews* 11 (November 14, 2012): CD001167, www.ncbi.nlm.nih.gov/pubmed/23152205.

30. N. A. Freasey, G. Dougan, R. A. Kingsley, et al., "Invasive Non-typhoidal Salmonella Disease: An Emerging and Neglected Tropical Disease in Africa," *Lancet* 379 (June 30, 2012): 2489–99, www.ncbi.nlm.nih.gov/pubmed/22587967.

31. WHO International Review Panel, "Impacts of Growth Promoter Termination," pp. 20–30; DANMAP 2003, pp. 34–35.

32. DANMAP 1997–2012; 1997, pp. 18–19; 1998, pp. 30–35; 1999, pp. 29–32; 2000, pp. 29–33; 2001, pp. 34–40; 2002, pp. 30–37; 2003, pp. 32–40; 2004, pp. 44–53; 2005, pp. 51–56; 2006, pp. 47–48, 54; 2012, data for figures with zoonotic and indicator bacteria, p. 74, fig. 7.1. *E. faecalis* erythromycin resistance also decreased: 53 percent in broiler chickens and 63 percent in pigs.

33. A. M. Hammerum, C. H. Lester, J. Neimann, et al., "A Vancomycin-Resistant Enterococcus faecium Isolate from a Danish Healthy Volunteer, Detected 7 Years after the Ban of Avoparcin, Is Possibly Related to Pig Isolates," *Journal of Antimicrobial Chemotherapy* 53 (2004): 547–49.

34. WHO International Review Panel, "Impacts of Growth Promoter Termination," pp. 20–30. There is cross reactivity between tylosin and erythromycin, since both are macrolide antibiotics.

35. DANMAP 1997–2007; 1997, pp. 18–19; 1998, pp. 30–35; 1999, pp. 29–32; 2000, pp. 29–33; 2001, pp. 34–40; 2002, pp. 30–37; 2003, pp. 32–40; 2004, pp. 44–53; 2005, pp. 51–56; 2006, pp. 47–48, 54; 2007, p. 59.

36. DANMAP 2010, p. 81.

37. DANMAP 2002, p. 39.

38. Hammerum et al., "Vancomycin-Resistant Enterococcus faecium Isolate." See also A. M. Hammerum, "Enterococci of Animal Origin and Their Significance for Public Health," *Clinical Microbiology and Infection* 18 (2012): 619–25. Therapeutic use of tetracycline could coselect for vancomycin resistance.

39. Hammerum, "Enterococci of Animal Origin."

40. Anette M. Hammerum, head, Antimicrobial Resistance Reference Laboratory, Department of Microbiology and Infection Control, Division of Microbiology and Diagnostics, Statens Serum Institut, e-mail communication, January 10, 2014. The role of microbes, including colonization with resistant organisms such as VRE, in the human gut is not well understood. A new field of medicine called the human microbiome is developing to study the interactions between microbes and human cells. S. Khanna and P. K. Tosh, "A Clinician's Primer on the Role of the Microbiome in Human Health and Disease," *Mayo Clinic Proceedings* 89 (January 2014): 107–14.

41. There is no enterococci data from primary care.

42. DANMAP 2008, p. 84; 2009, p. 84; 2010, p. 97; 2011, p. 110; 2012, p. 95; 2013, p. 85.

43. DANMAP 2007, p. 65; 2008, p. 84; 2010, p. 97; 2011, p. 110; 2012, p. 95. From 2002 to 2012, ampicillin resistance in *E. faecium* bacteremias increased 45 percent. See also Hammerum, e-mail communication, January 10, 2014. Genetic analysis suggests that *E. faecium* isolates from hospitalized patients belong to different genotypes than those isolated from animals or healthy humans.

44. DANMAP 2013, p. 86; *vanA* genes confer resistance to vancomycin.

45. DANMAP 2003, p. 23 (converted to DDD / 100 occupied bed-days); 2012, p. 54.

46. Cephalosporins are a class of b-lactam antibiotics, like penicillins. There are three generations of cephalosporins. The first generation is most effective against Gram-positive bacteria. Third-generation cephalosporins are more effective against Gram-negative bacteria. The second generation's activity is in between that of the first and the third.

47. DANMAP 2003, p. 23 (converted to 100 occupied bed-days); 2012, p. 54.

48. Maja Larsen, PhD, Drug Statistics Register, Sector for National Health Documentation and Research, Denmark, e-mail communications, November 20, December 19, 2013. However, while the length of stay decreased, the admission rate increased 23 percent.

49. DANMAP 2003, p, 21; 2012, p. 47.

50. DANMAP 2003, p. 21, table 13; 2012, p. 47, table 5.2.

51. European Centre for Disease Prevention and Control, "Summary of the Latest Data on Antibiotic Consumption in the European Union," November 2012, Stockholm, Sweden, p. 4, www.ecdc.europa.eu/en/eaad/documents/esac-net-summary-antibiotic-consumption .pdf.

52. Danish Health and Medicines Authority, "Guidelines on Prescribing Antibiotics," November 2013, Copenhagen, Denmark, http://sundhedsstyrelsen.dk/publ/Publ2013/11nov /AntibioPrescribDK_En.pdf. The guidelines were written in accordance with sec. 17 of the Consolidated Act No. 877 of August 4, 2011, on the authorization of health personnel and on professional health activities.

53. Ibid., p. 4.

54. European Centre for Disease Prevention and Control, "Antimicrobial Resistance Surveillance in Europe," 2012, Annual Report of the European Antimicrobial Resistance Surveillance Network (EARS-Net), Stockholm, Sweden, http://ecdc.europa.eu/en/publications/Publications /antimicrobial-resistance-surveillance-europe-2012.pdf. See also P. Collignon, F. M. Aarestrup, R. Irwin, et al., "Human Deaths and Third-Generation Cephalosporin Use in Poultry, Europe,"

Emerging Infectious Diseases 19 (2013): 1339–40, wwwnc.cdc.gov/eid/article/19/8/12-0681
_article.htm.

55. Collignon et al., "Human Deaths and Third-Generation Cephalosporin Use;
DANMAP 2012, p. 83.

56. WHO International Review Panel, "Impacts of Growth Promoter Termination," p. 7.

57. DANMAP 2004, p. 24, table 11.

58. Statistics 2013 Pigmeat, Landbrug Fødevarer (Danish agriculture and food council),
June 2014, "Structure of Suppliers in Denmark," p. 3, www.agricultureandfood.co.uk/
Statistics/Pig_industry_statistics.aspx.

59. DANMAP 2013, p. 21, table 3.1.

60. Statistics Denmark. Data obtained by e-mail from Pia Nielsen, senior health clerk,
External Economy, December 11, 2014.

61. FAOSTAT, "Exports: Countries by Commodities," http://faostat.fao.org/site/342/de
fault.aspx.

62. R. J. L. Willems, J. Top, W. van Schaik, et al., "Restricted Gene Flow among Hospital
Subpopulations of Enterococcus faecium," *mBio* 3, no. 4 (2012): e00151-12, doi: 10.1128/mBio
.00151-12, http://mbio.asm.org/content/3/4/e00151-12.abstract.

CHAPTER SIX: The European Experience

1. Quoted in M. Hornsby, "Farmers Fear Pounds 160M Cost of Antibiotic Ban," *London
Times,* December 4, 1998.

2. "Advisory Committee's Report on Microbial Antibiotic Resistance and Food Safety in
the United Kingdom," *Eurosurveillance* 3, no. 35 (August 26, 1999), www.eurosurveillance
.org/ViewArticle.aspx?ArticleId=1343.

3. J. Revill, "Epidemic Alert over `Superbugs' in British Meat," *London Evening Standard,*
August 18, 1999.

4. "EU to Ban Poultry Feed with Key Antibiotics," *Birmingham Post,* November 13, 1998.
Cattle feed made from infected sheep brains and nervous tissue led to the emergence of
bovine spongiform encephalopathy. See also M. Mann, "Europe: Plan for Total Ban on Antibiotics in Animal Feed: Food Safety Commission Says Products Used to Boost Growth in
Livestock Should Be Phased out by 2006," *Financial Times,* March 26, 2002.

5. G. Follet, "Antibiotic Resistance in the EU—Science, Politics, and Policy," *AgBioForum*
3 (2000): 148–55, www.agbioforum.org/v3n23/v3n23a13-follet.pdf. The 14 key resistant
pathogens in human medicine are Methicillin-resistant *Staphylococcus aureus* (MRSA), *Mycobacterium* tuberculosis, *Streptococcus* pneumonia, *Streptococcus pyogenes, Neisseria meningitides,
Neisseria* gonorrhea, *Campylobacter spp, Salmonella spp, E coli* (urogen, 0157), Vancomycin-
resistant *enterococci, Pseudomonas aeruginosa, Klebsiella spp, Acinetobacter spp,* and *Enterobac-
ter spp.* European Commission, Directorate-General XXIV, Consumer Policy and Consumer
Health Protection, Directorate B—Scientific Health Opinions, Unit B3—Management of
Scientific Committees II, "Opinion of the Scientific Steering Committee on Antimicrobial
Resistance," May 28, 1999, 22–35, http://ec.europa.eu/food/fs/sc/ssc/out50_en.pdf.

6. R. J. Bywater and M. W. Casewell, "An Assessment of the Impact of Antibiotic Resistance in Different Bacterial Species and of the Contribution of Animal Sources to Resistance
in Human Infections," *Journal of Antimicrobial Chemotherapy* 46 (2000): 639–45.

7. According to an ECDC–European Food Safety Authority (EFSA)–European Medicines
Agency (EMA) Joint Interagency Antimicrobial Consumption and Resistance Analysis Report, published on January 30, 2015, that analyzed consumption of antibiotics in humans
and food-producing animals in 26 EU or EEA countries in 2012, the average consumption
expressed as milligrams per kilogram of estimated biomass was 116.4 mg/kg in humans

(range 56.7–175.8) and 144.0 mg/kg in animals (range 3.8–396.5mg/kg), p. 29, www.ecdc .europa.eu/en/publications/Publications/antimicrobial-resistance-JIACRA-report.pdf.

8. Follet, "Antibiotic Resistance in the EU."

9. European Union Press Release, IP/02/1891, "Council Backs Prohibition of Antibiotics as Growth Promoters: Byrne Welcomes Political Agreement on Feed Additives," Brussels, December 16, 2002, europa.eu/rapid/press-release_IP-02-1891_en.pdf.

10. Mann, "Europe"; "EU to Ban Poultry Feed"; UNESCO, "The Precautionary Principle," World Commission on the Ethics of Scientific Knowledge and Technology, 2005, pp. 7–8, http://unesdoc.unesco.org/images/0013/001395/139578e.pdf. Rather than address risks *after* a crisis, the precautionary principle addresses risks *before* a crisis (anticipatory measures), even if the science is not fully understood. Some would argue, however, that this approach presents its own problems.

11. Commissioner Byrne, the former attorney general of Ireland, who wrote the amendments to the Irish Constitution that ended the conflict in Northern Ireland, was equally successful as the EU's first commissioner of health and consumer protection. During his tenure, from 1999 to 2004, Byrne established the European Food Safety Authority (EFSA), an independent institution that advised policymakers on risk assessments relating to food, and the European Centre for Disease Surveillance and Control (ECDC), which conducted coordinated surveillance of communicable diseases. Europe's Health Commissioner, "From the Good Friday Agreement to the Global Health Discussion," Metropolitan Corporate Counsel, October 1, 2004, Northeast Edition, www.metrocorpcounsel.com/articles/4639 /europes-health-commissioner-good-friday-agreement-global-health-discussion, p. 36; Mann, "Europe"; "EU to Ban Poultry Feed."

12. "EU to Ban Poultry Feed"; David Byrne, telephone interview, March 4, 2014. According to Byrne, the government in Belgium was up for reelection in 1999 when the dioxin scandal broke. The government, including the prime minister, was not reelected.

13. Influenced by the Swann Report, the European Economic Community passed Council Directive 70/524, December 14, 1970, which set basic standards for additives in animal feed; the member states had two years to bring their national rules and regulations into compliance with this directive. Council Directive 70/524 did not include any prohibitions on the use of antibiotics as growth promoters in animal feed. From 1973 to 1978, several annexes regarding the use of antibiotics in livestock were added to Council Directive 70/524. These annexes were limited in scope. Annex I listed antibiotics allowed in animal feeds without marketing restrictions; annex II listed antibiotics that could be used by member nations within their national jurisdictions. As new scientific data pertaining to antibiotic use in feeds became known, the annex lists were updated.

14. Regulation (EC) No. 1831/2003 of the European Parliament and of the Council, "On Additives for Use in Animal Nutrition," *Eur-Lex* (Access to European Union law), September 22, 2003, http://eur-lex.europa.eu/legal-content/en/TXT/?uri=CELEX:32003R1831; J. I. R. Castanon, "History of the Use of Antibiotic as Growth Promoters in European Poultry Feeds," *Poultry Science* 86 (2007): 2466–71, http://ps.fass.org/content/86/11/2466.full.pdf.

15. "Council Recommendation of 15 November 2001 on the Prudent Use of Antimicrobial Agents in Human Medicine (2002/77/EC)," *Official Journal of the European Communities,* 2002, http://eur-lex.europa.eu/LexUriServ/LexUriServ.do?uri=OJ:L:2002:034:0013:0016:EN:PDF.

16. Commission of the European Communities, "Report from the Commission to the Council. On the Basis of Member States' Reports on the Implementation of the Council Recommendation (2002/77/EC) on the Prudent Use of Antimicrobial Agents in Human Medicine," Brussels, Belgium, December 22, 2005, http://ec.europa.eu/health/ph_threats /com/mic_res/com684_en.pdf.

17. Ibid., pp. 3, 4. The countries providing this education were not listed in the first report.

18. European Commission, "Second Report from the Commission to the Council: On the Basis of Member States' Reports on the Implementation of the Council Recommendation (2002/77/EC) on the Prudent Use of Antimicrobial Agents in Human Medicine," April 9, 2010, pp. 3–5. http://ec.europa.eu/health/antimicrobial_resistance/docs/amr_report2_en .pdf.

19. Commission of the European Communities, Commission Staff Working Document, "Accompanying Document to the Second Report from the Commission to the Council on the Basis of Member States' Reports on the Implementation of the Council Recommendation (2002/77/EC) on the Prudent Use of Antimicrobial Agents in Human Medicine," April 9, 2010, pp. 16–17, http://ec.europa.eu/health/antimicrobial_resistance/docs/cswd_technicalannex_e n.pdf.

Countries reporting antibiotic sales without prescriptions	*Percentage of antibiotics sold without prescriptions*
Austria, Belgium, Czech Republic, Estonia, Italy, Netherlands, United Kingdom	Less than 1 percent
Bulgaria, Cyprus, Latvia, Lithuania, Poland	Between 1 and 5 percent
Malta, Romania, Spain	Between 5 and 10 percent
Greece	More than 15 percent
Portugal	Data missing

20. Ibid., p. 20; European Commission, "Second Report to the Council," p. 5.

21. European Commission, "Second Report to the Council," pp. 5–6. From 2001 to 2007, the European Commission's Directorate-General for Health and Consumers funded the University of Antwerp in Belgium to coordinate the ESAC-Net project that collected comparable data from publicly available sources on antimicrobial consumption in Europe. The European Centre for Disease Prevention and Control (ECDC) funded ESAC-Net from 2007 to 2011. Thirty-five countries voluntarily participated, including all EU member states, Iceland, Norway, Switzerland, Croatia, Turkey, Russia, the former Yugoslav Republic of Macedonia, and Israel. In July 2011, the project was transferred to the ECDC and became ESAC-Net. More detailed information on its history is available in the 2010 ESAC-Net report, p. 4, http://ecdc.europa.eu/en/publications/Publications/antimicrobial-antibiotic-consumption -ESAC-report-2010-data.pdf.

22. N. Adriaenssens, S. Coenen, A. Versporten, et al., "European Surveillance of Antimicrobial Consumption (ESAC): Outpatient Antibiotic Use in Europe (1997–2009)," *Journal of Antimicrobial Chemotherapy* 66, Suppl 6 (2011): vi3–vi12. The 35 countries include all 27 EU member states, 3 European Economic Area–European Free Trade Association (EEA–EFTA) countries (Iceland, Norway, and Switzerland), 3 candidate countries (Croatia, Macedonia, and Turkey), and 2 other countries (Russian Federation and Israel).

23. Adriaenssens et al., "European Surveillance of Antimicrobial Consumption"; ESAC Yearbook 2006, p. 37, table 3; ESAC Yearbook 2007, p. 39, table 3.3; ESAC Yearbook 2009, p. 43, table 3.3; 2011 Surveillance Report, p. 51, table 4.1, http://ecdc.europa.eu/en/activities /surveillance/ESAC-Net/publications/Pages/documents.aspx.

24. ECDC, "Surveillance Reports: Surveillance of Antimicrobial Consumption in Europe," http://ecdc.europa.eu/en/activities/surveillance/ESAC-Net/publications/Pages/documents

.aspx, 2011 Report, p. 11, table 3.1; ESAC Yearbook 2009, p. 35, table 3.1. Cyprus included both community and hospital antibiotic use in all reported years, and Greece included both from 2004 to 2008.

25. Ibid.; ESAC Yearbook 2009, p. 24, fig. 3.12. Data courtesy of ECDC TESSy Data Access Team, Surveillance of Antimicrobial Consumption in Europe: (a) Cyprus, Iceland, and Slovakia provided total care data (i.e., including the hospital sector); (b) Spain and Romania provided reimbursement data (i.e., not including consumption without a prescription and other nonreimbursed courses).

26. Data courtesy of ECDC TESSy Data Access Team, Surveillance of Antimicrobial Consumption in Europe. Some countries provided only consumption data in community settings and were not displayed; most vancomycin consumption was in hospitals.

27. N. Adriaenssens, S. Coenen, A. Versporten, et al., "European Surveillance of Antimicrobial Consumption (ESAC): Quality Appraisal of Antibiotic Use in Europe," *Journal of Antimicrobial Chemotherapy* 66, Suppl 6 (2011): vi71–vi77.

28. Gimenez Encarna, Data Access Team, ECDC, e-mail communication, April 10, 2014.

29. A. Kleinman, L. Eisenberg, and B. Good, "Clinical Lessons from Anthropologic and Cross-Cultural Research," *Annals of Internal Medicine* 88 (1978): 251–58; A. Zuger, "One Injury, 10 Countries: A Journey in Health Care," *New York Times,* September 15, 2009, www.nytimes.com/2009/09/15/health/15book.html. For example, recommended treatments for shoulder injuries can vary considerably from country to country.

30. European Medicines Agency, "First Report. Trends in the Sales of Veterinary Antimicrobial Agents in Nine European Countries," September 2011, p. 6, www.ema.europa.eu/ema/index.jsp?curl=pages/regulation/document_listing/document_listing_000302.jsp.

31. European Medicines Agency, "Trends in the Sales of Veterinary Antimicrobial Agents in Nine European Countries: Reporting Period: 2005–2009," September 15, 2011, www.ema.europa.eu/docs/en_GB/document_library/Report/2011/09/WC500112309.pdf. The nine countries were Czech Republic, Denmark, Finland, France, the Netherlands, Norway, Sweden, Switzerland, and the United Kingdom.

32. Ibid., pp. 7, 23, 26, 27, 33.

33. European Surveillance of Veterinary Antimicrobial Consumption (ESVAC), "Sales of Veterinary Antimicrobial Agents in 25 EU/EEA Countries in 2011," October 2013, p. 63, www.ema.europa.eu/ema/index.jsp?curl=pages/regulation/document_listing/document_listing_000302.jsp.

34. EU Directorate-General for Agriculture and Rural Development, "Agriculture in the European Union: Statistical and Economic Information 2011," March 2012, pp. 54–55, http://ec.europa.eu/agriculture/statistics/agricultural/2011/pdf/full-report_en.pdf.

35. European Surveillance, "Sales of Veterinary Antimicrobial Agents," p. 63.

36. Ibid. See also P. Collignon, F. M. Aarestrup, R. Irwin, et al., "Human Deaths and Third-Generation Cephalosporin Use in Poultry, Europe," *Emerging Infectious Diseases* 19 (2013): 1339–40, wwwnc.cdc.gov/eid/article/19/8/12-0681_article.htm.

37. European Surveillance, "Sales of Veterinary Antimicrobial Agents," p. 63.

38. Collignon et al., "Human Deaths and Third-Generation Cephalosporin Use"; I. Overdevest, I. Willemsen, M. Rijnsburger, et al., "Extended-Spectrum ß-Lactamase Genes of Escherichia coli in Chicken Meat and Humans, the Netherlands," *Emerging Infectious Diseases* 17 (2011): 1216–22, wwwnc.cdc.gov/eid/article/17/7/11-0209_article.htm.

39. Overdevest et al., "Extended-Spectrum ß-Lactamase Genes"; 2011 data from ESVAC shows that the Netherlands is the sixth-largest consumer of antibiotics in livestock behind Germany, Spain, Italy, France, and Poland. See also Collignon et al., "Human Deaths and Third-Generation Cephalosporin Use."

40. M. E. A. de Kraker, P. G. Davey, H. Grundmann, et al., "Mortality and Hospital Stay Associated with Resistant Staphylococcus aureus and Escherichia coli Bacteremia: Estimating the Burden of Antibiotic Resistance in Europe," *PLoS Medicine* 8 (2011): e1001104, http://journals.plos.org/plosmedicine/article?id=10.1371/journal.pmed.1001104.

41. Data-collection methodology is explained in the Annual Report of the European Antimicrobial Resistance Surveillance Network (EARS-Net), 2012, Country summary sheets, pp. 77–81, www.ecdc.europa.eu/en/publications/Publications/antimicrobial-resistance-surveillance-europe-2012.pdf. Antibiotic resistance data is collected from hospitals and laboratories.

42. Data derived from the Annual Report of EARS-Net, 2012, Country summary sheets, pp. 83–202.

43. Ibid.

44. Data from 2011 derived from Annual Report of EARS-Net, 2012. The 10 countries are Belgium, Denmark, France, Germany, Italy, Netherlands, Poland, Spain, Sweden, and the United Kingdom.

45. "EU Summary Report on Antimicrobial Resistance in Zoonotic and Indicator Bacteria from Humans, Animals and Food 2011," *EFSA Journal* 11, no. 5 (2013): 3196, p. 10, www.efsa.europa.eu/en/efsajournal/doc/3196.pdf; European Food Safety Authority (EFSA), Scientific Report of EFSA, "Technical Specifications on the Harmonized Monitoring and Reporting of Antimicrobial Resistance in Salmonella, Campylobacter and Indicator Escherichia coli and Enterococcus spp. bacteria Transmitted through Food," *EFSA Journal* 10, no. 6 (2012): 2742, p. 2, www.efsa.europa.eu/en/search/doc/2742.pdf.

46. "EU Summary Report on Antimicrobial Resistance," 203. The countries were Austria, Belgium, Denmark, Finland, France, Germany, Ireland, the Netherlands, Spain, Norway, and Switzerland.

47. The countries were Belgium, Denmark, France, Germany, the Netherlands, and Spain.

48. Koen Van Dyck, MD, MFH, head of unit, Health & Consumers Directorate General, Directorate G—Veterinary and International Affairs, e-mail communication, March 21, 2014. The other antibiotic feed additives that were banned in 1997 and 1998 were bacitracin zinc, spiramycin, virginiamycin, and tylosin phosphate. Four remaining antibiotics authorized for use as growth promoters (flavophospholipol, salinomycin sodium, avilamycin, and monesin sodium) belong to classes of compounds not used in human medicine.

49. "Annual Report of EARS-Net, 2013," Country summary sheets, pp. 83, 95, 103, 115, 119, 123, 135, 139, 159, 171, 187, 191, 195, www.ecdc.europa.eu/en/publications/Publications/antimicrobial-resistance-surveillance-europe-2013.pdf.

50. "Annual Report of EARS-Net, 2012," Country summary sheets, pp. 83–202.

51. I. Klare, D. Badstubner, C. Konstabel, et al., "Decreased Incidence of VanA-type Vancomycin-Resistant Enterococci Isolated from Poultry Meat and from Fecal Samples of Humans in the Community after Discontinuation of Avoparcin Usage in Animal Husbandry," *Microbial Drug Resistance* 5 (1999): 45–52; A. E. Van den Bogaard and E. E. Stobberingh, "The Effect of Banning Avoparcin on VRE Carriage in the Netherlands," *Journal of Antimicrobial Chemotherapy* 46 (2000): 145–53.

52. Van den Bogaard and Stobberingh, "Effect of Banning Avoparcin."

53. European Centre for Disease Prevention and Control (ECDC), "Antimicrobial Resistance Surveillance in Europe 2013," Annual Report of the European Antimicrobial Resistance Surveillance Network (EARS-Net). Stockholm: ECDC; 2014, http://ecdc.europa.eu/en/publications/Publications/antimicrobial-resistance-surveillance-europe-2013.pdf, pp. 87, 99, 123, 135, 139, 143, 151, 171, 175.

54. "EU Summary Report on Antimicrobial Resistance," pp. 240, 254, tables EN3 and EN6. Eight countries provided data either for broilers or for pigs: Austria, Belgium, Denmark, France, Ireland, the Netherlands, Spain, and Sweden.

55. FAO Stat: The Statistics Division of the FAO, http://faostat3.fao.org/download/Q /QL/E.

56. South America overtook Europe after 2008, but its performance is not relevant for this analysis.

57. FAO Stat: The Statistics Division of the FAO. The calculations were made by the author alone and do not represent the opinions of the FAO.

58. FAO Stat Production Data Item code 1035 (Hg=heclogram [100 grams]), http:// faostat3.fao.org/faostat-gateway/go/to/download/Q/QL/E.

59. FAO Stat Production Data Item, code 5424.

60. FAOSTAT: Exports. Countries by commodity, http://faostat.fao.org/site/342/default .aspx.

61. ECDC/EMA Technical Report, "The Bacterial Challenge: Time to React: A Call to Narrow the Gap between Multidrug-Resistant Bacteria in the EU and the Development of New Antibacterial Agents," 2009, Stockholm, Sweden, www.ecdc.europa.eu/en/publications /Publications/0909_TER_The_Bacterial_Challenge_Time_to_React.pdf. The seven bacteria are methicillin-resistant *S. aureus,* vancomycin-resistant *Staphylococcus aureus,* vancomycin-resistant *Enterococcus* (e.g., *E. faecium*), penicillin-resistant *Streptococcus pneumonia,* third-generation resistant *Enterobacteriaceae* (e.g., *E. coli* and *Klebsiella pneumonia*), carbapenem-resistant *Enterobacteriaceae* (e.g., *K. pneumoniae*), and carbapenem-resistant *P. aeruginosa.*

62. Ibid., pp. 13, 14, table 2.

63. ECDC/EMA Technical Report, "The Bacterial Challenge." Extra hospital days, additional deaths, and yearly economic burden from VRE and third-generation cephalosporin-resistant *E. coli* infections were derived from p. 14, table 2. See www.press.jhu.edu.

64. European Commission, Directorate-General for Health & Consumers, Communication from the Commission to the European Parliament and the Council, "Action Plan against the Rising Threats from Antimicrobial Resistance," November 15, 2011, Brussels, Belgium, http://ec.europa.eu/dgs/health_consumer/docs/communication_amr_2011_748_en.pdf.

CHAPTER SEVEN: The Controversy in the United States

1. R. A. Merrill, "Food Safety Regulation: Reforming the Delaney Clause," *Annual Review of Public Health* 18 (1997): 313–40, http://aseh.net/teaching-research/teaching-unit-better -living-through-chemistry/historical-sources/lesson-2/Merrill-Food percent20Safety percent-20Regulation-1997.pdf.

2. J. Akst, "The Elixir Tragedy, 1937," *Scientist,* June 1, 2013, www.the-scientist.com/?arti cles.view/articleNo/35714/title/The-Elixir-Tragedy--1937/.

3. Merrill, "Food Safety Regulation"; Penicillin Amendment of 1945, chap. 281, sec. 3, 59 Stat., pp. 463–64; L. Heinzerling, "Conference on Agriculture and Food Systems: September 28, 2012: Undue Process at the FDA: Antibiotics, Animal Feed, and Agency Intransigence," *Vermont Law Review* 37 (Summer 2013): 1007.

4. Heinzerling, "Conference on Agriculture and Food Systems." See also *Federal Register* 3647, 3648 (April 28, 1951); and *Federal Register* 2335 (April 22, 1953).

5. Merrill, "Food Safety Regulation."

6. S. B. Levy, *The Antibiotic Paradox: How Miracle Drugs Are Destroying the Miracle* (New York: Plenum Press, 1992), pp. 141–43, 241–42.

7. "Antibiotics Used in Veterinary Medicine and for Nonmedical Purposes: Required Data," *Federal Register,* chap. 1, part 3, sec. 3.55, 31, no. 163 (August 23, 1966).

8. "Food Safety and Quality: Use of Antibiotics in Animal Feed," part 2, 98-519, *Hearings before the Subcommittee on Agricultural Research and General Legislation*, 95th Cong., 1st Sess., September 21–22, 1977, p. 6.

9. Dr. C. D. VanHouweling, former director, Bureau of Veterinary Medicine (1969–79), interview by Ronald T. Ottes, June 18, 1990, Pella, Iowa, pp. 6–7, Department of Health and Human Services, Transcripts of the History of the U.S. Food and Drug Administration, www .fda.gov/downloads/AboutFDA/WhatWeDo/History/OralHistories/SelectedOralHistory Transcripts/UCM264576.pdf.

10. "Regulation of Food Additives and Medicated Animal Feeds," 62-868, *Hearings before a Subcommittee of the Committee on Government Operations*, 92nd Cong., 1st Sess., March 18, 1971, pp. 332–82.

11. "Food Safety and Quality."

12. Ibid., p. 5.

13. Ibid., pp. 7, 9. During the hearing, Edward J. Allera, associate chief counsel for veterinary medicine, Office of General Counsel, provided the statutory citation for Kennedy's statements. According to Allera, "The Animal Drug Amendments of 1968 were a consolidation of the Food Additive Amendments of 1958 and the Drug Amendments of 1962. They were added in 1968 to consolidate into one statutory section the separate statutory provisions covering premarket approval of chemicals intended for use in food-producing animals and for chemical additives to animals. FDA uses the basic safety standards that apply to food additives [that are] applicable to saccharin. We assess the risk and eschew the benefits in the risk calculation" (p. 9).

14. Ibid., pp. 35–36. David A. Phillipson, DVM, president of Animal Health Institute, and vice president of Upjohn Co., Kalamazoo, MI, commented on the FDA's regulatory policies:

> We are currently hamstrung by the Bureau of Veterinary Medicine and the Food and Drug Administration. The combination drug policy was developed . . . for human usage. And the agency has taken the same principle and attempted to apply it to animal husbandry and animal agriculture. We are not dealing with humans. We never will have an animal-rearing system that even compares to the treatment of humans. We have about 6,500 veterinarians who have to take care of some 4 billion food animals and fowl, which is a very high ratio of animals to veterinarians. We feel that when you have large confined flocks of 10,000 to 30,000 birds, or you have a 100,000 head feedlot, that you cannot diagnose and treat each of them individually because you probably have a multitude of organisms that are prevalent in this sort of population. . . . We feel very strongly that the FDA needs to undertake a very critical review of its combination drug policy and develop one that is appropriate for animal agriculture. (p. 40)

According to Bernadette Dunham, DVM, PhD, director of the Center for Veterinary Medicine, U.S. Food and Drug Administration, in an e-mail communication, May 9, 2014:

> Drugs intended for use in food-producing animals must be safe for both the target animals (the animals to whom the drug is administered) and for people eating food derived from the treated animals. Prior to the 1968 Animal Drug Amendments to the Federal Food, Drug, and Cosmetic Act, animal drugs were reviewed under two different statutory provisions and required approval under both section 505 (drug approval) and section 409 (food additive approval). In 1968, the Federal Food, Drug, and Cosmetic Act was amended to consolidate these provisions in a new section 512 of the Act. When we review a drug intended for a food-producing animal under sec-

tion 512, we look at the safety of the drug to the target animal (the animal receiving the drug) and the safety of the drug to humans consuming food from the treated animal. The standard for the target animal safety evaluation involves assessing the risks and benefits to the target animal. The standard for the human food safety evaluation involves determining whether there is a "reasonable certainty of no harm" to humans consuming food from animals treated with the drug. We do not look at benefits when assessing the human food safety of the drug.

15. "Food Safety and Quality," p. 27.

16. Ibid., pp. 38, 39.

17. Ibid., pp. 51, 55–56.

18. VanHouweling interview, p. 9.

19. Office of Technology Assessment, "Drugs in Livestock Feed," NITS order PB-298450, June 1979, pp. 5–7, http://ota.fas.org/technology_assessment_and_congress/.

20. Ibid., p. 8.

21. Ibid., pp. 11–13.

22. "Significant Dates in U.S. Food and Drug Law History," US FDA website, www.fda.gov/AboutFDA/WhatWeDo/History/Milestones/ucm128305.htm; *Hearings before the Subcommittee on Investigations and Oversight of the Committee on Science and Technology,* U.S. House of Representatives, 98th Cong., 2nd Sess., December 18, 19, 1984, 43-016, p. 2.

23. R. A. Merrill, "FDA's Implementation of the Delaney Clause: Repudiation of Congressional Choice or Reasoned Adaptation to Scientific Progress?" *Yale Journal on Regulation* 5 (1988): 1–88; Food and Drug Administration, "Diethylstilbestrol: Withdrawal of Approval of New Animal Applications; Commissioner's Decision," *Federal Register* 44 (1979): 54852–900.

24. National Research Council, "The Effects on Human Health of Subtherapeutic Use of Antimicrobials in Animal Feeds," National Academies, Washington, DC, 1980, 53, www.nap.edu/openbook.php?record_id=21&page=53.

25. Levy, *Antibiotic Paradox;* "Our History," Alliance for the Prudent Use of Antibiotics website, www.tufts.edu/med/apua/about_us/history.shtml.

26. "Our History." See also D. Barboza and S. Day, "McDonald's Seeking Cut in Antibiotics in its Meat," *New York Times,* June 20, 2003, www.nytimes.com/2003/06/20/business/mcdonald-s-seeking-cut-in-antibiotics-in-its-meat.html?module=Search&mabReward=relbias%2C%5B%22RI%3A9%22%2C%22RI%3A12%22%5D.

27. Barboza and Day, "McDonald's Seeking Cut."

28. FDA, Advisory Committees, VMAC Transcript, May 10, 1995, Archived Document, pp. 34–37; Pat McDermott, director of NARMS, FDA, e-mail communication, July 10, 2014. The FDA Veterinary Medical Advisory Committee was terminated on September 24, 2013. Dept. of HHS, 21 CFR Part 14, p. 6991, *Federal Register* 78, no. 226 (November 22, 2013), www.gpo.gov/fdsys/pkg/FR-2013-11-22/pdf/2013-27854.pdf. According to Laura Bradford, FDA, Center for Veterinary Medicine, Office of Director, Education and Outreach, the FDA was using the VMAC only sporadically and decided that there were better ways to discuss topics with new technologies; the meetings were not the best use of resources. www.fda.gov/AdvisoryCommittees/CommitteesMeetingMaterials/VeterinaryMedicineAdvisoryCommittee/.

29. General Accounting Office (GAO), "Antibiotic Resistance: Agencies Have Made Limited Progress Addressing Antibiotic Use in Animals," September 2011, GAO-11-801, p. 15, www.gao.gov/new.items/d11801.pdf.

30. Pat McDermott, e-mail communication, July 10, 2014.

31. CDC, National Antimicrobial Resistance Monitoring System, "About NARMS, Tracking Trends in Resistance," www.cdc.gov/narms/about/index.html.

32. U.S. Department of Agriculture, Agricultural Research Service, "NARMS Overview," www.ars.usda.gov/Main/docs.htm?docid=6750.

33. FDA, NARMS, "2009 Executive Report, Methods," pp. 4–5, www.fda.gov/downloads /AnimalVeterinary/SafetyHealth/AntimicrobialResistance/NationalAntimicrobialResistanc eMonitoringSystem/UCM268954.pdf.

34. Ibid., p. 17. Ten states are in the CDC's FoodNet program: Connecticut, Georgia, Maryland, Minnesota, New Mexico, Oregon, Tennessee, and various counties in California, Colorado, and New York. Pennsylvania volunteered to participate, as well. The surveillance area includes about 48 million people (approximately 15% of the US population). CDC, "About FoodNet," www.cdc.gov/foodnet/about.html.

35. CDC, "Salmonella, Diagnosis and Treatment," www.cdc.gov/salmonella/general/diag nosis.html.

36. USDA, NARMS, "Animal Arm," www.ars.usda.gov/SP2UserFiles/Place/66120508/NA RMS/percent_resistance/SalmChickenSlaughter.pdf; FDA, NARMS Report 2011, p. 23, table 8, www.fda.gov/downloads/AnimalVeterinary/SafetyHealth/AntimicrobialResistance/National AntimicrobialResistanceMonitoringSystem/UCM334834.pdf; USDA, NARMS, www.ars.usda .gov/SP2UserFiles/Place/66120508/NARMS/%_resistance/SalmSwineSlaughter.pdf; CDC, NARMS Annual Report 2011, p. 31, table 8, www.cdc.gov/narms/pdf/2011-annual-report -narms-508c.pdf.

37. CDC, "Campylobacter," www.cdc.gov/nczved/divisions/dfbmd/diseases/campylobacter /#treat.

38. USDA, 1998–2004, www.ars.usda.gov/SP2UserFiles/Place/66120508/CampyResist Summary98-04.pdf; USDA, 2005–2010, www.ars.usda.gov/SP2UserFiles/Place/66120508 /CampyResistSummary05-09.pdf; FDA, NARMS Report 2011, p. 40, table 16, www.fda.gov /downloads/AnimalVeterinary/SafetyHealth/AntimicrobialResistance/NationalAntimicrobi alResistanceMonitoringSystem/UCM334834.pdf; CDC, NARMS Annual Report 2011, p. 56, table 50, www.cdc.gov/narms/pdf/2011-annual-report-narms-508c.pdf.

39. C. S. Wong, J. Srdjan, R. L. Habeeb, et al., "The Risk of the Hemolytic-Uremic Syndrome after Antibiotic Treatment of Escherichia coli O157:H7 Infections," *New England Journal of Medicine* 342 (2000): 1930–36, www.nejm.org/doi/full/10.1056/nejm200006293422601; C. S. Wong, J. C. Mooney, J. R. Brandt, et al., "Risk Factors for the Hemolytic Uremic Syndrome in Children Infected with Escherichia coli O157:H7: A Multivariable Analysis," *Clinical Infectious Diseases* 55 (2012): 33–41, doi: 10.1093/cid/cis299, http://cid.oxfordjournals.org/content /early/2012/05/02/cid.cis299.short.

40. CDC, NARMS Annual Report 2011, p. 53, table 43.

41. USDA, NARMS, www.ars.usda.gov/SP2UserFiles/Place/66120508/NARMS/percent_re sistance/E.coli-RSummary.pdf; FDA, NARMS Report 2011, p. 60, table 26; CDC, NARMS Annual Report 2011, p. 53, table 43.

42. FDA, NARMS Report 2011, p. 60, table 26.

43. USDA, NARMS, Annual Animal Report 2011, pp. 16, 52, table 4D. The enterococcus isolates from chickens were "unspecified species." The isolates from chicken meat and pork chops were *Enterococcus faecium* and *Enterococcus faecalis*. www.ars.usda.gov/SP2UserFiles/Place /66120508/NARMS/NARMS2011/NARMS%20USDA%202011%20Report.pdf; FDA, NARMS Report 2011, pp. 50–51, tables 22.1 and 22.2.

44. L. C. McDonald, S. Rossiter, C. Mackinson, et al., "Quinupristin-Dalfopristin-Resistant Enterococcus Faecium on Chicken and in Human Stool Specimens," *New England Journal of Medicine* 345 (2001): 1155–60, www.nejm.org/doi/pdf/10.1056/NEJMoa010805.

45. J. Edelsberg, D. Weycker, R. Barron, et al., "Prevalence of Antibiotic Resistance in U.S. Hospitals," *Diagnostic Microbiology and Infectious Disease* 78 (2014): 255–62, www.ncbi.nlm .nih.gov/pubmed/24360267; CDC, "Antibiotic Resistance Threats in the United States 2013," p. 67, www.cdc.gov/drugresistance/threat-report-2013/pdf/ar-threats-2013-508.pdf.

46. L. C. McDonald, M. J. Kuehnert, F. C. Tenover, et al., "Vancomycin-Resistant Entero-cocci Outside the Health-Care Setting: Prevalence, Sources, and Public Health Implica-tions," *Emerging Infectious Diseases* 3 (1997): 311–17, wwwnc.cdc.gov/eid/article/3/3/97-0307 _article.

47. C. A. Arias and B. E. Murray, "The Rise of the Enterococcus: Beyond Vancomycin Re-sistance," *Nature Reviews Microbiology* 10 (April 2012): 266–78, www.nature.com/nrmicro /journal/v10/n4/pdf/nrmicro2761.pdf.

48. J. Top, R. Willems, and M. Bonten, "Emergence of CC17 Enterococcus faecium: From Commensal to Hospital-adapted Pathogen," *FEMS Immunology and Medical Microbiology* 52 (2008): 297–308.

49. R. Willems and W. van Schaik, "Transition of *Enterococcus faecium* from Commensal Organism to Nosocomial Pathogen," *Future Microbiology* 4 (2009): 1125–35. The United States has experienced two waves of resistant enterococci: the first, involving *E. faecalis,* in the late 1970s, was associated with the introduction of third-generation cephalosporins, and the second, involving *E. faecium,* in the early 1990s, was associated with the increased use of vancomycin and broad-spectrum antibiotics.

50. Willems and van Schaik, "Transition of *Enterococcus faecium.*"

51. Ibid.

52. P. Damborg, A. H. Sorensen, and L. Guardabassi, "Monitoring of Antimicrobial Re-sistance in Healthy Dogs: First Report of Canine Ampicillin-resistant *Enterococcus faecium* Clonal Complex 17," *Veterinary Microbiology* 132 (2008): 190–96; P. Damborg, J. Top, A. P. Hendrickx, et al., "Dogs Are a Reservoir of Ampicillin-Resistant *Enterococcus faecium* Lineages Associated with Human Infections," *Applied and Environmental Microbiology* 75 (2009): 2360–65.

53. Damborg et al., "Dogs Are a Reservoir." Dog samples came from two longitudinal studies: one involving families with humans and their healthy companion dogs and the other involving sick dogs with pyoderma (a skin infection) that were being treated with dif-ferent antibiotics (e.g., amoxicillin-clavulanic acid, cefovecin, and cephalexin).

54. USDA, Animal and Plant Health Inspection Service (APHIS), "A 40-Year Retrospec-tive of APHIS, 1972–2012," pp. 28, 29, https://www.aphis.usda.gov/about_aphis/downloads /40_Year_Retrospective.pdf.

55. Dr. Lonnie King, e-mail communication, July 18, 2014.

56. USDA, Animal and Plant Health Inspection Service, National Animal Health Monitor-ing System (NAHMS) website, www.aphis.usda.gov/wps/portal/aphis/home/?1dmy&urile =wcm%3apath%3a%2Faphis_content_library%2Fsa_our_focus%2Fsa_animal_health%2Fsa _monitoring_and_surveillance%2Fsa_nahms%2Fct_national_animal_health_monitoring _system_nahms_home.

57. USDA, APHIS, "Salmonella on U.S. Swine Sites—Prevalence and Antimicrobial Suscep-tibility," January 2009, table 3, www.aphis.usda.gov/animal_health/nahms/swine/downloads /swine2006/Swine2006_is_salmonella.pdf.

58. Eric J. Bush, veterinary epidemiologist, Animal and Plant Health Inspection Service, USDA, personal communication, January 20, 2015.

59. USDA, APHIS, "Campylobacter on U.S. Swine Sites—Antimicrobial Susceptibility," December 2008, table 1, www.aphis.usda.gov/animal_health/nahms/swine/downloads /swine2006/Swine2006_is_campy.pdf.

60. Eric J. Bush, personal communication, January 20, 2015.

61. USDA, APHIS, "Escherichia coli on U.S. Swine Sites—Antimicrobial Drug Suscepti-bility." January 2009, table 1, www.aphis.usda.gov/animal_health/nahms/swine/downloads/swine2006/Swine2006_is_ecoli.pdf.

62. USDA, APHIS, "Commensal Enterococcus on U.S. Swine Sites: Prevalence and Anti-microbial Drug Susceptibility," April 2009. Enterococcus species included *E. hirae* (29.6%), *E. faecalis* (27.4%), *E.* species not identified (16%), *E. faecium* (7.9%), *E. mundtii* (7.7%), *E. cas-seliflavus* (3%), and others. hwww.aphis.usda.gov/animal_health/nahms/swine/downloads/swine2006/Swine2006_is_entero.pdf; Eric J. Bush, personal communication, January 20, 2015.

63. S. M. Donabedian, M. B. Perri, N. Abdujamilova, et al., "Characterization of Vancomycin-Resistant Enterococcus faecium Isolated from Swine in Three Michigan Coun-ties," *Journal of Clinical Microbiology* 48 (2010): 4156–60. Fecal samples were obtained from 158 humans, 55 pigs, 50 cattle, 25 horses, 57 sheep, 14 goats, and 1 llama.

64. D. Vallenet, L. Labarre, Z. Rouy, et al., "MaGe: A Microbial Genome Annotation Sys-tem Supported by Synteny Results," *Nucleic Acids Research* 34 (2006): 53–65, www.ncbi.nlm.nih.gov/pubmed/16407324.

65. CDC, "Antibiotic Resistance Threats," pp. 6, 11, extrapolated from R. R. Roberts, B. Hota, I. Ahmad, et al., "Hospital and Societal Costs of Antimicrobial-resistant Infections in a Chicago Teaching Hospital: Implications for Antibiotic Stewardship," *Clinical Infectious Diseases* 49, no. 8 (2009): 1175–84.

66. CDC, "Antibiotic Resistance Threats," p. 7.

67. CDC, "Antibiotic Resistance Threats," pp. 65–67, 15–17, 65.

68. Ibid., p. 71.

69. R. L. Scharff, "Economic Burden from Health Losses Due to Foodborne Illness in the United States," *Journal of Food Protection* 75 (2012): 123–31, table 4, col. 3.

70. GAO, "Antibiotic Resistance," p. 11; FDA, "FDA Solicits Comments Related to the Collection of Sales and Distribution Data of Antimicrobial Animals Drugs," www.fda.gov/AnimalVeterinary/NewsEvents/CVMUpdates/ucm313294.htm.

71. FDA, "Antimicrobial Animal Drug Distribution Reports 2009–2011," www.fda.gov/ForIndustry/UserFees/AnimalDrugUserFeeActADUFA/ucm042896.htm. Antibiotics in the "NIR" category were not independently reported. The drug classes included aminocouma-rins, glycolipids, pleuromutilins, polypeptides, and quinoxalines.

72. FDA, "Antimicrobial Animal Drug Distribution Reports," p. 40, table 10, www.fda.gov/downloads/ForIndustry/UserFees/AnimalDrugUserFeeActADUFA/UCM416983.pdf.

73. USDA, APHIS, "Disease in Nursery and Grower/Finisher Pigs in 2000 and 2006—and Vaccine and Antimicrobial Use in 2006," January 2008, www.aphis.usda.gov/animal_health/nahms/swine/downloads/swine2006/Swine2006_is_nurserydis.pdf.

74. USDA, "Veterinary Services Factsheet: Antibiotic Usage in Premarket Swine," Janu-ary 1996, www.aphis.usda.gov/animal_health/nahms/swine/downloads/swine95/Swine95_is_antib.pdf.

75. USDA, APHIS, "Info Sheet: Disease Prevention, Treatment Practices, and Antibiotic Ad-ministration Techniques on U.S. Swine Sites," table 1, www.aphis.usda.gov/animal_health/nahms/swine/downloads/swine2006/Swine2006_is_DisPrev.pdf. Data represented 94 percent of US pig producers with 100 or more pigs, representing 94 percent of the total US pig inventory.

76. M. D. Apley, E. J. Bush, R. B. Morrison, et al., "Use Estimates of In-Feed Antimicrobi-als in Swine Production in the United States," *Foodborne Pathogens and Disease* 9 (2012):

272–79, table 5, col. 1, www.nppc.org/wp-content/uploads/Swine-in-feed-use-estimates .pdf.

77. Suraj Pant, research analyst, Center for Disease Dynamics, Economics & Policy, "Outpatient Antibiotic Use," http://cddep.org/projects/resistance_map/outpatient_antibi-otic_use; L. A. Hicks, T. H. Taylor, and R. J. Hunkler, "U.S. Outpatient Antibiotic Prescribing, 2010," *New England Journal of Medicine* 368 (2013): 1461–62.

78. Hicks, Taylor, and Hunkler, "U.S. Outpatient Antibiotic Prescribing."

79. T. P. Van Boeckel, S. Gandra, A. Ashok, et al., "Global Antibiotic Consumption 2000 to 2010: An Analysis of National Pharmaceutical Sales Data," *Lancet Infectious Diseases* 14 (2014): 742–50, www.thelancet.com/journals/laninf/article/PIIS1473-3099(14)70780-7/full text#article_upsell.

80. H. A. Kirst, D. G. Thompson, and T. I. Nicas, "Historical Yearly Usage of Vancomy-cin," *Antimicrobial Agents and Chemotherapy* 42 (1998): 1303–4, www.ncbi.nlm.nih.gov/pmc /articles/PMC105816/.

81. Willems and van Schaik, "Transition of *Enterococcus faecium.*"

82. B. McKay and V. Bauerlein, "CDC: Antibiotic Overuse Can Be Lethal," *Wall Street Journal,* March 4, 2014, http://online.wsj.com/news/articles/SB100014240527023045850045 79419493198620498.

83. Hicks, Taylor, and Hunkler, "U.S. Outpatient Antibiotic Prescribing"; Dr. Stuart B. Levy, professor of molecular biology, microbiology, and medicine, Tufts University School of Medi-cine, director of the Center for Adaptation Genetics and Drug Resistance, president of the Alli-ance for the Prudent Use of Antibiotics, telephone interview by the author, July 23, 2014.

84. J. Perry, D. E. Banker, and R. Green, "Poultry Production in the United States," Broiler Farms' Organization, Management, and Performance, AIB-748, March 1999, USDA Economic Research Service, p. 1, www.ers.usda.gov/media/256034/aib748b_1_.pdf. The per-centage of farms raising chickens has been falling since the 1920s, but the methodology of calculating them changed after 1969. So only the data since 1969 is given. USDA, National Agricultural Statistics Service, Charts and Maps, "Broilers: Inventory by State, US," www .nass.usda.gov/Charts_and_Maps/Poultry/brlmap.asp.

85. USDA, National Agricultural Statistics Service, Charts and Maps, "Hogs: Number of Operations by Year, US," www.nass.usda.gov/Charts_and_Maps/Hogs_and_Pigs/hgoper _e.asp.

86. USDA, National Agricultural Statistics Service, Charts and Maps, "Meat Animals: Production by Year," www.nass.usda.gov/Charts_and_Maps/Meat_Animals_PDI/lbspr.asp.

87. USDA, National Agricultural Statistics Service, Charts and Maps, "Broilers: Produc-tion by Year, US," www.nass.usda.gov/Charts_and_Maps/Poultry/brlprd.asp.

88. USDA, Economic Research Service, "Outbreak of Porcine Epidemic Diarrhea Virus (PEDv) Impacts Forecast of 2014 U.S. Pork Output," www.ers.usda.gov/data-products/chart-gallery/detail .aspx?chartId=43866; K. Gee, "Futures Prices Are Going Hog-wild," *Wall Street Journal,* March 5, 2014, www.wsj.com/articles/SB10001424052702304732804579421613265579806.

89. B. Mole, "Deadly Pig Virus Slips through U.S. Borders," *Nature* 499 (2013), doi:10 .1038/499388a; K. Gee, "Pork Prices Drop as Hog Herds Recover," *Wall Street Journal,* Janu-ary 26, 2015, www.wsj.com/articles/pork-prices-drop-as-hog-herds-recover-1422307742.

90. USDA, Economic Research Service, "Hogs & Pork. Trade," www.ers.usda.gov/topics /animal-products/hogs-pork/trade.aspx.

91. USDA, Economic Research Service, "Food Availability (per Capita) Data System: Red Meat (beef, veal, pork, lamb, and mutton)," www.ers.usda.gov/data-products/food-avail ability-%28per-capita%29-data-system.aspx.

92. USDA, Economic Research Service, "Food Availability (per Capita) Data System: Poultry (chicken and turkey)," www.ers.usda.gov/data-products/food-availability-%28per -capita%29-data-system.aspx.

93. David Harvey, USDA Economic Research Service, personal communication, June 27, 2014.

94. USDA, Economic Research Service, "Food Availability: Poultry"; U.S. Census Bureau, Foreign Trade, www.census.gov/foreign-trade/statistics/highlights/top/top1411yr.html. The top 15 countries the United States exports to are Canada, Mexico, China, Japan, United Kingdom, Germany, South Korea, Netherlands, Brazil, Hong Kong, Belgium, France, Singapore, Australia, and Taiwan.

95. USDA, Economic Research Service, "Meat Price Spreads," including historical monthly price spread data for beef, pork, broilers; retail prices for beef, pork, poultry cuts, eggs, and dairy products; and pork values and spreads, www.ers.usda.gov/data-products/meat -price-spreads.aspx; and U.S. Dept. of Labor, Bureau of Labor Statistics, Consumer Price Index, Data Tools, Databases, Tables, & Calculators by Subject, http://data.bls.gov/cgi-bin /surveymost?ap. Poultry includes chicken, turkey, duck, and quail. For pork: Consumer Price Index, All Urban Consumers, US City Average, http://data.bls.gov/pdq/querytool.jsp ?survey=cu.

96. USDA, Economic Research Service, "Food Availability: Poultry" (chicken and turkey); "Food Availability: Red Meat" (beef, pork, lamb, and mutton), retail meat pounds per US population per year.

97. International Labor Organization, LABORSTA. Note: UK 1991 price, Consumer Price Indices, Main statistics annual, laborsta.ilo.org/STP/guest.

98. S. L. Gorbach, "Antimicrobial Use in Animal Feed—Time to Stop," *New England Journal of Medicine* 345 (2001): 1202–3.

99. H.R. 962 (110th Cong.), Preservation of Antibiotics for Medical Treatment Act of 2007, www.govtrack.us/congress/bills/110/hr962; H.R. 1549 (111th Cong.), H.R. 965 (112th Cong.), H.R. 1150 (113th Cong.).

100. S. Tavernise, "Farm Use of Antibiotics Defies Scrutiny," *New York Times,* September 3, 2012, www.nytimes.com/2012/09/04/health/use-of-antibiotics-in-animals-raised-for-food -defies-scrutiny.html?pagewanted=all; M. McKenna, "Antibiotic Overuse on Farms: Is the Opinion Tide Turning?" *Wired,* November 4, 2013, www.wired.com/2013/11/antibiotic -opinion-turning/; L. Sayre, "The Hidden Health Hazards of Factory Farms," *Mother Earth News,* February–March 2009, www.motherearthnews.com/natural-health/health-hazards -factory-farms-zmaz09fmzraw.aspx#axzz38s9UJyAD.

101. L. Zuraw, "Ruling on FDA's Oversight of Animal Antibiotic Use Called a `Big Blow to Public Health,'" *Food Safety News,* July 25, 2014, www.foodsafetynews.com/2014/07 /appeals-court-rules-fda-not-required-to-hold-hearings-on-animal-antibiotic-use/# .U9eqFv2jShM.

102. G. Harris, "Steps Set for Livestock Antibiotic Ban," *New York Times,* March 23, 2012, www.nytimes.com/2012/03/24/health/fda-is-ordered-to-restrict-use-of-antibiotics-in -livestock.html?scp=1&sq=judge%20theodore%20h.%20katz&st=cse.

103. FDA, "Guidance for Industry on the Judicious Use of Medically Important Antimicrobial Drugs in Food-Producing Animals: Availability," April 13, 2012, www.fda.gov /downloads/AnimalVeterinary/GuidanceComplianceEnforcement/GuidanceforIndustry /UCM216936.pdf; FDA, "FDA Takes Steps to Protect Public Health," News and Events, April 11, 2012, www.fda.gov/NewsEvents/Newsroom/PressAnnouncements/ucm299802 .htm.

104. Richard Carnevale, VMD, vice president, Regulatory, Scientific, and International Affairs, Animal Health Institute, Washington DC, telephone interview by the author, September 3, 2014.

105. G. Harris, "U.S. Tightens Rules on Antibiotics Use for Livestock," *New York Times,* April 11, 2012, www.nytimes.com/2012/04/12/us/antibiotics-for-livestock-will-require-pres cription-fda-says.html; Zuraw, "Ruling on FDA's Oversight"; R. Reichl, "The FDA's Blatant Failure on Food," *New York Times,* July 30, 2014, www.nytimes.com/2014/07/31/opinion/the -fda-blatant-failure-on-food.html.

106. White House, "National Strategy for Combating Antibiotic Resistant Bacteria," September 2014, www.whitehouse.gov/sites/default/files/docs/carb_national_strategy.pdf; The American Presidency Project, Barack Obama, XLIV President of the United States, 677 Executive Order 13676—Combating Antibiotic-Resistant Bacteria, September 18, 2014, www.presidency.ucsb.edu/ws/index.php?pid=107546; John Woolley, professor of political science and codirector of the American Presidency Project, University of California, Santa Barbara, e-mail communication, January 30, 2015, www.presidency.ucsb .edu/. According to Woolley, no executive order since 1945 contained the phrase "antibiotic resistance." President Obama neither cited an authority nor referred to prior executive orders. President Carter issued an executive order that dealt with the export of "uncertified" antibiotics.

107. Executive Office of the President, President's Council of Advisors on Science and Technology, "Report to the President on Combating Antibiotic Resistance," September 2014, www.whitehouse.gov/sites/default/files/microsites/ostp/PCAST/pcast_carb_report_sept 2014.pdf.

108. White House Office of the Press Secretary, "Fact Sheet: President's 2016 Budget Proposes Historic Investment to Combat Antibiotic-Resistant Bacteria to Protect Public Health," January 27, 2015, www.whitehouse.gov/the-press-office/2015/01/27/fact-sheet-president-s -2016-budget-proposes-historic-investment-combat-a.

109. S. A. Miller and S. Dinan, "Obama, Democrats Clash with New GOP Majority as 114th Congress Convenes," *Washington Times,* January 6, 2015, www.washingtontimes.com /news/2015/jan/6/obama-democrats-clash-with-new-republican-majority/?page=all.

CHAPTER EIGHT: International Challenges

1. World Health Organization, Drug Resistance, *WHO Global Strategy for Containment of Antimicrobial Resistance,"* www.who.int/drugresistance/WHO_Global_Strategy.htm/en/.

2. WHO, *Global Strategy for Containment of Antimicrobial Resistance* (Geneva: World Health Organization Press, 2001), www.who.int/drugresistance/WHO_Global_Strategy_English.pdf; Fifty-First World Health Assembly, WHA51.17, Agenda item 21.3, "Emerging and Other Communicable Diseases: Antimicrobial Resistance," May 16, 1988, http://apps.who.int/medi cinedocs/index/assoc/s16334e/s16334e.pdf?ua=1.

3. WHO, "Mobilizing Political Will to Contain Antimicrobial Resistance," *Bulletin of the World Health Organization* 89 (2011): 168–69, www.who.int/bulletin/volumes/89/3/11 -030311/en/.

4. WHO, *Global Strategy for Antimicrobial Resistance.*

5. WHO, "Mobilizing Political Will."

6. D. Yong, M. A. Toleman, C. G. Giske, et al., "Characterization of a New Metallo-β-Lactamase Gene, *bla*$_{NDM-1}$, and a Novel Erythromycin Esterase Gene Carried on a Unique Genetic Structure in *Klebsiella pneumonia* Sequence Type 14 from India," *Antimicrobial Agents and Chemotherapy* 53 (2009): 5046–54.

7. K. K. Kumarasamy, M. A. Toleman, T. R. Walsh, et al., "Emergence of a New Antibiotic Resistance Mechanism in India, Pakistan, and the U.K.: A Molecular, Biological, and Epidemiological Study," *Lancet Infectious Diseases* 10 (2010): 597–602, www.ncbi.nlm.nih.gov/pmc/articles/PMC2933358/.

8. WHO, *Antimicrobial Resistance: Global Report on Surveillance 2014* (Geneva: World Health Organization Press, 2014), www.who.int/drugresistance/documents/surveillancereport/en/.

9. P. Stephens, "Antibiotic Resistance Now `Global Threat,' WHO Warns," *BBC News Health,* April 30, 2014, www.bbc.com/news/health-27204988; C. Larano, "Antibiotic Resistance a Major Public Health Threat, WHO Report Confirms," *Wall Street Journal,* Southeast Asia, May 1, 2014, http://blogs.wsj.com/indonesiarealtime/2014/05/01/antibiotic-resistance-a-major-public-health-threat-who-report-confirms/.

10. WHO, *Antimicrobial Resistance;* ibid., pp. 9, 10.

11. Ibid., pp. xi, 59–62. *E. coli* causes urinary tract and bloodstream infections in hospitals and communities. Nontyphoidal *Salmonella* causes foodborne diarrhea and bloodstream infections in the community. The 11 countries are Canada, Denmark, Finland, France, Germany, Japan, Norway, Italy, Netherlands, United States, and Sweden. See also F. M. Aarestrup, *Antimicrobial Resistance in Bacteria of Animal Origin* (Washington, DC: ASM Press, 2006), p. 406. This book lists 13 countries that collect data: Denmark, Belgium, Canada, France, Hungary, Italy, Japan, the Netherlands, Norway, Spain, Sweden, United Kingdom, and United States. Denmark was the first to establish its surveillance system, in 1995; the United States was second, in 1996.

12. WHO, Global Foodborne Infections Network (GFN), "Strategic Plan 2011–2015," www.who.int/entity/gfn/publications/strategic_plan_2011/en/index.html.

13. WHO, *Antimicrobial Resistance,* p. 61.

14. Ibid., annex 2, pp. 77–96. Levy described a study in 1969 finding resistant *E. coli* from one indigenous person and resistant unspecified bacteria from a soil specimen from the Solomon Islands. In the early 1960s, these findings were not common in environments where antibiotics had never been introduced. S. Levy, *The Antibiotic Paradox: How Miracle Drugs Are Destroying the Miracle* (New York: Plenum Press, 1992), pp. 74–75.

15. WHO, *Antimicrobial Resistance,* annex 2, pp. 128–35.

16. T. P. Van Boeckel, S. Gandra, A. Ashok, et al., "Global Antibiotic Consumption 2000 to 2010: An Analysis of National Pharmaceutical Sales Data," *Lancet Infectious Diseases* 14 (2014): 742–50, www.thelancet.com/journals/laninf/article/PIIS1473-3099(14)70780-7/fulltext#article_upsell. The finding that Germany is a high user of cephalosporins and fluoroquinolones contradicts ECDC findings as discussed in chapter 6. Greece and Cyprus were high consumers of all antibiotics including cephalosporins, but their consumption rates combined both outpatient clinic and hospital data. Germany, however, is a very high user of both tetracyclines and penicillins in livestock.

17. J. Carlet, V. Jarlier, S. Harbarth, et al., "Ready for a World without Antibiotics? The Pensieres Antibiotic Resistance Call to Action," *Antimicrobial Resistance and Infection Control* 1 (2012): 11, www.aricjournal.com/content/1/1/11.

18. D. J. Morgan, I. N. Okeke, R. Laxminarayan, et al., "Non-prescription Antimicrobial Use Worldwide: A Systematic Review," *Lancet Infectious Diseases* 11 (2011): 692–701, www.sciencedirect.com/science/article/pii/S1473309911700548.

19. S. Rowbotham, A. Chisholm, and S. Moschogianis, "Challenges to Nurse Prescribers of a No-antibiotic Prescribing Strategy for Managing Self-Limiting Respiratory Tract Infections," *Journal of Advanced Nursing* 68 (2012): 2622–32, http://onlinelibrary.wiley.com/doi/10.1111/j.1365-2648.2012.05960.x/full.

20. R. S. Saver, "In Tepid Defense of Population Health: Physicians and Antibiotic Resistance," *American Journal of Law & Medicine* 34 (2008): 431–91.

21. WHO, "Mobilizing Political Will"; F. L. Bavestrello and M. A. Cabello, "Community Antibiotic Consumption in Chile, 2000–2008," *Revista Chilena de infectologia* 28 (2011): 107–12, http://europepmc.org/abstract/MED/21720688. Public education was an integral part of the effort, but one study has shown that knowledge alone does not necessarily change behavior. C. A. M. McNulty, P. Boyle, T. Nichols, et al., "Don't Wear Me Out—The Public's Knowledge of and Attitudes to Antibiotic Use," *Journal of Antimicrobial Chemotherapy* 59 (2007): 727–38, http://jac.oxfordjournals.org/content/59/4/727.full.

22. McNulty et al., "Don't Wear Me Out." Other Chilean industries include copper mining, forestry products, and wine. A. Barrionuevo, "Chile's Antibiotics Use on Salmon Farms Dwarfs That of a Top Rival's," *New York Times,* July 27, 2009, www.nytimes.com/2009/07/27/world/americas/27salmon.html.

23. A. Barrionuevo, "Salmon Virus Indicts Chile's Fishing Methods," *New York Times,* March 27, 2008, www.nytimes.com/2008/03/27/world/americas/27salmon.html?pagewanted=all; A. H. Buschmann, A. Tomova, and A. Lopez, "Salmon Aquaculture and Antimicrobial Resistance in the Marine Environment," *PLOS ONE* 7 (8): e42724, doi: 10.1371/journal.pone.0042724, www.plosone.org/article/info%3Adoi%2F10.1371%2Fjournal.pone.0042724.

24. A. Barrionuevo, "Chile under Fire for Results of Intensive Salmon Fish Farms," *New York Times,* March 26, 2008, www.nytimes.com/2008/03/26/health/26iht-salmon.4.11444981.html?pagewanted=all.

25. A. Faiz and A. Basher, "Antimicrobial Resistance: Bangladesh Experience," *Regional Health Forum (SEARO)* 15 (2011): 1–8, www.searo.who.int/publications/journals/regional_health_forum/media/2011/V15n1/rhfv15n1p1.pdf.

26. S. Kariuki, the Global Antibiotic Resistance Partnership—Kenya National Working Group, "Situation Analysis and Recommendations: Antibiotic Use and Resistance in Kenya," Center for Disease Dynamics, Economics & Policy, August 2011, pp. 4–7, www.cddep.org/publications/situation_analysis_and_recommendations_antibiotic_use_and_resistance_kenya.

27. A. Syed Rehan, A. Shakeel, and L. Heeramani, "Trends of Empiric Antibiotic Usage in a Secondary Care Hospital, Karachi, Pakistan," *International Journal of Pediatrics* (2013), Article ID 832857, www.hindawi.com/journals/ijpedi/2013/832857/.

28. F. Qazi, N. Bano, SadiaZafar, et al., "Self-Medication of Antibiotics in Pharyngitis and Gastroenteritis—A Community Based Study in Karachi, Pakistan," *International Journal Pharmaceutical Sciences Review and Research* 21 (2013): 207–11, http://globalresearchonline.net/journalcontents/v21-2/38.pdf.

29. Q. A. Shah, D. J. Colquhoun, H. L. Kijuli, et al., "Prevalence of Antibiotic Resistance Genes in the Bacterial Flora of Integrated Fish Farming Environments of Pakistan and Tanzania," *Environmental Science & Technology* 46 (2012): 8672–79, http://pubs.acs.org/doi/abs/10.1021/es3018607.

30. M. Idrees, M. Ali Shah, S. Michael, et al., "Antimicrobial Resistant Escherichia coli Strains Isolated from Food Animals in Pakistan," *Pakistan Journal of Zoology* 43 (2011): 303–10, http://zsp.com.pk/303-310%20(13)%20PJZ-368-10.pdf.

31. Ibid.

32. V. J. Wirtz, A. Dreser, and R. Gonzales, "Trends in Antibiotic Utilization in Eight Latin American Countries, 1997–2007," *Revista Panamericana Salud Publica* 27 (2010): 219–25, www.scielosp.org/pdf/rpsp/v27n3/a09v27n3.pdf. The eight countries are Argentina, Brazil, Chile, Colombia, Mexico, Peru, Uruguay, and Venezuela.

33. Morgan et al., "Non-prescription Antimicrobial Use Worldwide"; L. Ecker, T. J. Ochoa, M. Vargas, et al., "Factors Affecting Caregiver's Use of Antibiotics Available without

a Prescription in Peru," *Pediatrics* 131 (2013): e1171, http://pediatrics.aappublications.org /content/131/6/e1771.full.pdf.

34. L. E. Redding, F. Cubas-Delgado, M. S. Sammel, et al., "The Use of Antibiotics on Small Dairy Farms in Rural Peru," *Preventive Veterinary Medicine* 113 (2014): 88–95, www .ncbi.nlm.nih.gov/pubmed/24188819.

35. United Nations Population Division, "India Becomes a Billionaire: World's Largest Democracy to Reach One Billion Persons on Independence Day," www.un.org/esa /population/pubsarchive/india/ind1bil.htm; Editorial Board, "India and the Post-antibiotic Era," *New York Times,* December 8, 2014, www.nytimes.com/2014/12/09/opinion/india-and -the-post-antibiotic-era.html?module=Search&mabReward=relbias%3Ar%2C%7B%221%22 %3A%22RI%3A5%22%7D.

36. G. Harris, "Poor Sanitation in India May Afflict Well-Fed Children with Malnutri-tion," *New York Times,* July 13, 2014, www.nytimes.com/2014/07/15/world/asia/poor-sanita-tion-in-india-may-afflict-well-fed-children-with-malnutrition.html; D. Coffey, A. Gupta, P. Hathi, et al., "Revealed Preference for Open Defecation: Evidence from a New Survey in Rural North India," SQUAT Working Paper No. 1, Rice Institute, June 26, 2014, http://squatreport .in/wp-content/uploads/2014/06/SQUAT-research-paper.pdf.

37. G. Harris, " 'Superbugs' Kill India's Babies and Pose an Overseas Threat," *New York Times,* December 3, 2014, www.nytimes.com/2014/12/04/world/asia/superbugs-kill-indias -babies-and-pose-an-overseas-threat.html?module=Search&mabReward=relbias%3Ar%2C %7B%221%22%3A%22RI%3A5%22%7D, derived from quote by Ramanan Laxminarayan, vice president for research and policy at the Public Health Foundation of India.

38. Global Antibiotic Resistance Partnership—India Working Group, "Rationalizing An-tibiotic Use to Limit Antibiotic Resistance in India," *Indian Journal of Medical Research* 134 (2011): 281–94, www.ncbi.nlm.nih.gov/pmc/articles/PMC3193708/; R. S. Sharma, S. M. Kaul, and J. Sokhay, "Seasonal Fluctuations of Dengue Fever Vector, Aedes Aegypti (Diptera: Culicidae) in Delhi, India," *Southeast Asian Journal of Tropical Medicine and Public Health* 36 (2005): 186–90; A. K. Hati, "Dengue Serosurveillance in Kolkata, Facing an Epidemic in West Bengal, India," *Journal of Vector Borne Diseases* 46 (2009): 197–204.

39. Global Antibiotic Resistance Partnership—India Working Group, "Rationalizing An-tibiotic Use."

40. D. N. Jha, "Stop Prescribing Antibiotics for Fever and Cold, Indian Medical Associa-tion Will Tell Doctors," *Times of India,* September 27, 2014, http://timesofindia.indiatimes .com/india/Stop-prescribing-antibiotics-for-fever-and-cold-Indian-Medical-Association-will -tell-doctors/articleshow/43569276.cms.

41. K. Sinha, "In a First, Antibiotics Bar on Food-Producing Animals," *Times of India,* April 6, 2012, http://timesofindia.indiatimes.com/india/In-a-first-antibiotics-bar-on-food -producing-animals/articleshow/12552605.cms; Global Antibiotic Resistance Partnership— India Working Group, "Rationalizing Antibiotic Use."

42. UN Food and Agriculture Organization, "Food and Nutrition in Numbers 2014: Rome, Italy," p. 30, www.fao.org/3/a-i4175e.pdf; Government of India, Ministry of Home Affairs, Office of the Registrar General and Census Commissioner, 2001 Census Data, Reli-gion, table 21, "Distribution of Population by Religion," http://censusindia.gov.in/(S(ajfapx 450hzqdpvhx2wl5au3))/Census_And_You/religion.aspx; P. Esselborn, "Vegetarians Develop-ing a Taste for Meat," *Deutsche Welle,* February 1, 2013, www.dw.de/vegetarians-developing -a-taste-for-meat/a-16490496; Y. Yadav and S. Kumar, "The Food Habits of a Nation," *Hindu,* August 14, 2006, www.thehindu.com/todays-paper/article3089973.ece.

43. National Dairy Development Board, "Milk Production in India," www.nddb.org /English/Statistics/Pages/Milk-Production.aspx. Launched in 1970 as Operation Flood, the

NDDB is an NGO dedicated to increasing milk production in rural areas. S. K. Narula, "India's 75 Million Dairy Farms Now Produce More Milk Than All of the European Union," *Quartz,* July 15, 2014, http://qz.com/235085/india-75-million-dairy-farms-now-make-more-milk -than-all-of-the-european-union/; Government of India, Ministry of Agriculture 16th & 19th Indian Livestock Census, 16th: chap. 2, pp. 2, 6; 19th: table 3.2, p. 15, http://dahd.nic .in/dahd/statistics/livestock-census.aspx.

44. J. Shaohong, "Regulations, Realities and Recommendations on Antimicrobial Use in Food Animal Productions in China," in *Medical Impact of Antimicrobial Use in Food Animals* (Geneva: WHO, 1997), chap. 9, pp. 91–92, http://apps.who.int/iris/bitstream/10665/64439/2 /WHO_EMC_ZOO_97.4_(WP1-22).pdf.

45. Y.-G. Zhu, T. A. Johnson, J.-Q. Su, et al. "Diverse and Abundant Antibiotic Resistance Genes in Chinese Swine Farms," *Proceedings of the National Academy of Sciences* 110 (2013): 3435–40, www.pnas.org/content/110/9/3435.full.pdf+html?sid=2b4b8e42-984c-4c4b-982f -490772ac2730; M. Hvistendahl, "China Takes Aim at Rampant Antibiotic Resistance," *Science* 336 (2012): 795; F. H. Wang, "The Estimation of the Production and Amount of Animal Manure and Its Environmental Effect in China," *China Environmental Science* 26 (2006): 614–17.

46. Zhu et al., "Diverse and Abundant Antibiotic Resistance"; R. Wei, F. Ge, S. Huang, et al., "Occurrence of Veterinary Antibiotics in Animal Wastewater and Surface Water around Farms in Jiangsu Province, China," *Chemosphere* 82 (2011): 1408–14, www.sciencedirect.com /science/article/pii/S0045653510013755; L. Zhao, Y. Hua Dong, and H. Wang, "Residues of Veterinary Antibiotics in Manures from Feedlot Livestock in Eight Provinces of China," *Science of the Total Environment* 408 (2010): 1069–75, www.sciencedirect.com/science/article/pii /S0048969709011036; X. Zhang, Y. Li, B. Liu, et al., "Prevalence of Veterinary Antibiotics and Antibiotic Resistant Escherichia coli on the Surface Water of a Livestock Production Region in Northern China," *PLOS ONE* 9 (2014): e111026. www.ncbi.nlm.nih.gov/pmc/articles/PMC 4220964/pdf/pone.0111026.pdf.

47. P.-L. Ho, E. Lai, P.-Y. Chan, et al., "Rare Occurrence of Vancomycin-Resistant Enterococcus faecium among Livestock Animals in China," *Journal of Antimicrobial Chemotherapy* 2013, doi: 10.1093/jac/dkt293; K. Tanimoto, T. Nomura, H. Hamatani, et al., "A Vancomycin-dependent VanA-type Enterococcus faecalis Strain Isolated in Japan from Chicken Imported from China," *Letters in Applied Microbiology* 41 (2005): 157–62. The strains were KC122.1 and KC122.3. KC122.1 was unusual in that it could grow only in the presence of glycopeptide in culture media—it was dependent on the presence of vancomycin to grow. It was a VanA-type VRE with high-level resistance to vancomycin. KC122.3 was able to grow with or without the presence of vancomycin. Japan used avoparcin between 1989 and 1996, but VRE had not been isolated from domestic chicken meat.

48. ST6 and CC5 are acronyms for Sequence Type 6 and Clonal Complex 5. These are terms used in epidemiological typing using DNA genetic analyses. Ho et al., "Rare Occurrence." See also A. R. Freitas, T. M. Coque, C. Novais, et al., "Human and Swine Hosts Share Vancomycin-Resistant *Enterococcus faecium* CC17 and CC5 and *Enterococcus faecalis* CC2 Clonal Clusters Harboring TN*1546* on Indistinguishable Plasmids," *Journal of Clinical Microbiology* 49 (2011): 925–31, table 2, doi: 10.1128/JCM.01750-10.

49. Food and Agriculture Organization, National Aquaculture Sector Overview, "China," www.fao.org/fishery/countrysector/naso_china/en.

50. Food and Agriculture Organization, Fisheries, Technical Paper 469, "Responsible Use of Antibiotics in Aquaculture," Rome, Italy, 2005, p. 23, table 3.5, www.fao.org/3/a-a0282e .pdf; S. Zou, W. Xu, R. Zhang, et al., "Occurrence and Distribution of Antibiotics in Coastal Water of the Bohai Bay, China: Impacts of River Discharge and Aquaculture Activities,"

Environmental Pollution 159 (2011): 2913–20, www.sciencedirect.com/science/article/pii /S0269749111002454; Q. Zheng, R. Zhang, Y. Wang, et al., "Occurrence and Distribution of Antibiotics in the Beibu Gulf, China: Impacts of River Discharge and Aquaculture Activities," *Marine Environmental Research* 78 (2012): 26–33, www.sciencedirect.com/science /article/pii/S0141113612000670.

51. Y. Li, "China's Misuse of Antibiotics Should Be Curbed," *British Medical Journal* 348 (2014): g1083, www.bmj.com/content/348/bmj.g1083; A. Heddini, O. Cars, S. Qiang, et al., "Antibiotic Resistance in China—A Major Future Challenge," *Lancet* 373 (2009): 30.

52. X. Yin, F. Song, Y. Gong, et al., "A Systematic Review of Antibiotic Utilization in China," *Journal of Antimicrobial Chemotherapy* 68 (2013): 2445–52.

53. J. Wang, P. Wang, X. Wang, et al., "Use and Prescription of Antibiotics in Primary Health Care Settings in China," *Journal of the American Medical Association Internal Medicine* 174 (2014): 1914–20, www.ncbi.nlm.nih.gov/pubmed/25285394.

54. Ibid. The Chinese Ministry of Health based its 2004 "Principles of Clinical Use of Antibiotics" on internationally endorsed criteria specified in I. C. Gyssens, P. J. Van Den Broek, B.-J. Kullberg, et al., "Optimizing Antimicrobial Therapy: A Method for Antimicrobial Drug Use Evaluation," *Journal of Antimicrobial Chemotherapy* 30 (1992): 724–27. Criteria for appropriate or inappropriate assessments of antibiotic prescriptions included whether sufficient data was available for proper diagnosis, dosage, dosage interval, route of administration, length of administration, and whether there was a better treatment option available. See also Y. Xiao and L. Li, "Legislation of Clinical Antibiotic Use in China," *Lancet* 13 (2013): 189–90.

55. Wang et al., "Use and Prescription of Antibiotics."

56. L. Reynolds and M. McKee, "Factors Influencing Antibiotic Prescribing in China: An Exploratory Analysis," *Health Policy* 90 (2009): 32–36; J. Currie, W. Lin, and J. Meng, "Addressing Antibiotic Abuse in China: An Experimental Audit Study," *Journal of Development Economics* 110 (2014): 39–51; Li, "China's Misuse of Antibiotics"

57. Currie, Lin, and Meng, "Addressing Antibiotic Abuse in China."

58. Y. Xiao, J. Zhang, B. Zheng, et al., "Changes in Chinese Policies to Promote the Rational Use of Antibiotics," *PLOS Medicine* 10 (2013): e1001556, doi: 10:10.1371/journal. pmed.1001556, www.plosmedicine.org/article/info%3Adoi%2F10.1371%2Fjournal.pmed.1001 556p; Li, "China's Misuse of Antibiotics"; Hvistendahl, "China Takes Aim."

59. Y.-H. Xiao, C. G. Giske, Z.-Q. Wei, et al., "Epidemiology and Characteristics of Antimicrobial Resistance in China," *Drug Resistance Updates* 14 (2011): 236–50.

60. Xiao et al., "Changes in Chinese Policies"; Xiao and Li, "Legislation of Antibiotic Use."

61. H. Sun, H. Wang, Y. Xu, et al., "Molecular Characterization of Vancomycin-Resistant Enterococcus Spp.: Clinical Isolates Recovered from Hospitalized Patients among Several Medical Institutions in China," *Diagnostic Microbiology and Infectious Disease* 74 (2012): 399–403. See also J. Top, R. Willems, and M. Bonten, "Emergence of CC17 Enterococcus faecium: From Commensal to Hospital-adapted Pathogen," *FEMS Immunology and Medical Microbiology* 52 (2008): 297–308, http://onlinelibrary.wiley.com/doi/10.1111/j.1574-695X.2008.00383 .x/abstract.

62. Xiao et al., "Changes in Chinese Policies."

63. Hvistendahl, "China Takes Aim"; Xiao and Li, "Legislation of Antibiotic Use."

64. Xiao et al., "Changes in Chinese Policies."

65. Ibid.

CHAPTER NINE: Environmental and Pharmaceutical Discoveries and Challenges

1. For example, J.-M. Monier, S. Demaneche, T. O. Delmont, et al., "Metagenomic Exploration of Antibiotic Resistance in Soil," *Current Opinion in Microbiology* 14 (2011): 229–35.

2. J. A. Perry and G. D. Wright, "The Antibiotic Resistance `Mobilome': Searching for the Link between Environment and Clinic," *Frontiers in Microbiology* 4 (2013): 1–7, http://journal.frontiersin.org/Journal/10.3389/fmicb.2013.00138/full; S. J. Salter, M. J. Cox, E. M. Turek, et al., "Reagent and Laboratory Contamination Can Critically Impact Sequence-based Microbiome Analyses," *BMC Biology* 12 (2014): 87, www.biomedcentral.com/1741 -7007/12/87.

3. J. F. Linares, I. Gustafsson, F. Baquero, et al., "Antibiotics as Intermicrobial Signaling Agents Instead of Weapons," *Proceedings of the National Academy of Sciences* 103 (2006): 19484–489, www.pnas.org/content/103/51/19484.full. See also J. L. Martinez, "Antibiotics and Antibiotic Resistance Genes in Natural Environments," *Science* 321 (2008): 365–67.

4. J. Nesme, S. Cecillon, T. O. Delmont, et al., "Large-Scale Metagenomic-Based Study of Antibiotic Resistance in the Environment," *Current Biology* 24 (2014): 1096–1100. See also B. Liu and M. Pop, "ARDB—Antibiotic Resistance Genes Database," *Nucleic Acids Research* 37 (2009): Database issue: D443–D447, http://nar.oxfordjournals.org/content/37/suppl_8/28 /15443.abstract.

5. Liu and Pop, "ARDB." Annotated reads are matching ARGD sequences found in the Antibiotic Resistance Genes Database (i.e., no evidence of effective resistance is shown with this sequence-base method).

6. V. M. D'Costa, C. E. King, L. Kalan, et al., "Antibiotic Resistance Is Ancient," *Nature* 477 (2011): 457–61; B. Steven, R. Leveille, W. H. Pollard, et al., "Microbial Ecology and Biodiversity in Permafrost," *Extremophiles* 10 (2006): 259–67.

7. C. W. Knapp, J. Dolfing, P. A. I. Ehlert, et al., "Evidence of Increasing Antibiotic Resistance Gene Abundances in Archived Soils since 1940," *Environmental Science and Technology* 44 (2010): 580–87.

8. Microbial transfer of genetic material can occur in three ways: (1) bacterial conjugation: through direct cell-to-cell contact via a pillus (tube); genetic material in the form of a plasmid (a circle of DNA) gets passed from one microbe to another; (2) transformation: a microbe takes up genetic material from a dead microbe that has released its contents into the environment; (3) transduction: genetic material is transferred from one bacterium to another by a bacteriophage (special virus).

9. H. Heuer, H. Schmitt, and K. Smalla, "Antibiotic Resistance Gene Spread Due to Manure Application on Agricultural Fields," *Current Opinion in Microbiology* 14 (2011): 236–42.

10. A CAFO is defined as a facility that raises animals in a confined setting for 45 days or more during a 12-month period and brings feed to the animals rather than has them graze or seek feed.

11. GAO, "Concentrated Animal Feeding Operations: EPA Needs More Information and a Clearly Defined Strategy to Protect Air and Water Quality from Pollutants of Concern," September 2008, GAO-08-944, p. 5, www.gao.gov/assets/290/280229.pdf.

12. Ibid., pp. 14, 18. Large hog farms were estimated to produce more than 15,000 tons, and broiler chicken farms were estimated to produce more than 6,400 tons of manure each year. The GAO used USDA data on large farms to estimate the number, size, and location of CAFOs, because no federal agency collects data on them.

13. M. F. Davis, L. B. Price, and C. M.-H. Liu, "An Ecological Perspective on U.S. Industrial Poultry Production: The Role of Anthropogenic Ecosystems on the Emergence of Drug-

Resistant Bacteria from Agricultural Environments," *Current Opinion in Microbiology* 14 (2011): 244–50.

14. Y. Yang, B. Li, S. Zou, et al., "Fate of Antibiotic Resistance Genes in Sewage Treatment Plant Revealed by Metagenomic Approach," *Water Research* 62 (2014): 97–106, www .sciencedirect.com/science/article/pii/S0043135414003728#.

15. E. M. H. Wellington, A. B. A. Boxall, P. Cross, et al., "The Role of the Natural Environment in the Emergence of Antibiotic Resistance in Gram-Negative Bacteria," *Lancet Infectious Disease* 13 (2013): 155–65.

16. K. Kummerer and A. Henninger, "Promoting Resistance by the Emission of Antibiotics from Hospitals and Households into Effluent," *Clinical Microbiology and Infection* 9 (2003): 1203–14.

17. F. C. Cabello, "Heavy Use of Prophylactic Antibiotics in Aquaculture: A Growing Problem for Human and Animal Health and for the Environment," *Environmental Microbiology* 8, no. 7 (2006): 1137–44; R. Goldburg and R. Naylor, "Future Seascapes, Fishing, and Fish Farming," *Frontiers in Ecology and the Environment* 3 (2005): 21–28.

18. Food and Agriculture Organization (FAO), "State of the World Fisheries and Aquaculture: Opportunities and Challenges," 2014, Rome, Italy, p. 19, www.fao.org/3/a-i3720e .pdf.

19. Cabello, "Heavy Use of Prophylactic Antibiotics"; H. Y. Done and R. U. Halden, "Reconnaissance of 47 Antibiotics and Associated Microbial Risks in Seafood Sold in the United States," *Journal of Hazardous Materials* 282 (2015): 10–17, http://dx.doi.org/10.1016/j.jhazmat .2014.08.075; T. Defoirdt, P. Sorgeloos, and P. Bossier, "Alternatives to Antibiotics for the Control of Bacterial Disease in Aquaculture," *Current Opinion in Microbiology* 14 (2011): 215–58.

20. C. S. Smillie, M. B. Smith, J. Friedman, et al., "Ecology Drives a Global Network of Gene Exchange Connecting the Human Microbiome," *Nature* 480 (2011): 241–44; K. J. Forsberg, A. Reyes, B. Wang, et al., "The Shared Antibiotic Resistome of Soil Bacteria and Human Pathogens," *Science* 337 (2012): 1107–11; G. Dantas and M. O. A. Sommer, "Context Matters—The Complex Interplay between Resistome Genotypes and Resistance Phenotypes," *Current Opinion in Microbiology* 15 (2012): 577–82.

21. D. I. Andersson and D. Hughes, "Antibiotic Resistance and Its Cost: Is It Possible to Reverse Resistance?" *Nature* 8 (2010): 260–71; D. I. Andersson and B. R. Levin, "The Biological Cost of Antibiotic Resistance," *Current Opinion in Microbiology* 2 (1999): 489–93.

22. S. J. Schrag and V. Perrot, "Reducing Antibiotic Resistance," *Nature* 381 (1996): 120–21; M. Sundqvist, P. Geli, D. I. Andersson, et al., "Little Evidence for Reversibility of Trimethoprim Resistance after a Drastic Reduction in Trimethoprim Use," *Journal of Antimicrobial Chemotherapy* 65 (2010): 350–60; V. I. Enne, D. M. Livermore, P. Stephens, et al., "Persistence of Sulphonamide Resistance in Escherichia coli in the UK despite National Prescribing Restriction," *Lancet* 357 (2001): 1325–28; M. Sjolund, K. Wreiber, D. I. Andersson, et al., "Long-Term Persistence of Resistant Enterococcus Species after Antibiotics to Eradicate Helicobacter pylori," *Annals of Internal Medicine* 139 (2003): 483–88.

23. Penicillin is typically the drug of choice for group A streptococcal (*Streptococcus pyogenes*) infections. Erythromycin is used in penicillin-allergic individuals. H. Seppala, T. Klaukka, J. Vuopio-Varkila, et al., "The Effect of Changes in the Consumption of Macrolide Antibiotics on Erythromycin Resistance in Group A Streptococci in Finland," *New England Journal of Medicine* 337 (1997): 441–46.

24. M. W. Climo, D. S. Israel, E. S. Wong, et al., "Hospital-Wide Restriction of Clindamycin: Effect on the Incidence of Clostridium difficile–Associated Diarrhea and Cost," *Annals of Internal Medicine* 128, no. 12, part 1 (1998): 989–95.

25. J. J. Rahal, C. Urban, D. Horn, et al., "Class Restriction of Cephalosporin Use to Control Total Cephalosporin Resistance in Nosocomial Klebsiella," *Journal of the American Medical Association* 280 (1998): 1233–37. The authors noted that all of the imipenem-resistant *P. aeruginosa* isolates, with one exception, remained susceptible to other β-lactam antibiotics, quinolones, or aminoglycosides. They concluded that their findings represented an overall reduction in nosocomial multiresistant gram-negative pathogens.

26. F. Bager, F. M. Aarestrup, M. Madsen, et al., "Glycopeptide Resistance in Enterococcus faecium from Broilers and Pigs Following Discontinued Use of Avoparcin," *Microbial Drug Resistance* 5 (1999): 53–56. Recall that avoparcin and vancomycin are both glycopeptide antibiotics. Resistance is mediated by the *van*A gene, which is located on a transposon, a DNA sequence that can change its position within a genome. A. E. van den Bogaard, N. Bruinsma, and E. E. Stobberingh, "The Effect of Banning Avoparcin on VRE Carrieage in the Netherlands," *Journal of Antimicrobial Chemotherapy* 46 (2000): 146–48.

27. I. Klare, D. Badstubner, C. Konstabel, et al., "Decreased Incidence of VanA-type Vancomycin-resistant Enterococci Isolated from Poultry Meat and from Fecal Samples of Humans in the Community after Discontinuation of Avoparcin Usage in Animal Husbandry," *Microbial Drug Resistance* 5 (1999): 45–52.

28. Wellington et al., "Role of the Natural Environment"; M. A. Gilliver, M. Bennett, M. Begon, et al., "Antibiotic Resistance Found in Wild Rodents," *Nature* 410 (1999): 233–34; I. Literak, M. Dolejska, T. Radimersky, et al., "Antimicrobial-Resistant Faecal Escherichia coli in Wild Mammals in Central Europe: Multiresistant Escherichia coli Producing Extended-Spectrum Beta-lactamases in Wild Boars," *Journal of Applied Microbiology* 108 (2010): 1702–11; T. Radimersky, P. Frolkova, D. Janoszowska, et al., "Antibiotic Resistance in Faecal Bacteria (Escherichia coli, Enterococcus spp.) in Feral Pigeons," *Journal of Applied Microbiology* 109 (2010): 1687–95; D. Costa, P. Poeta, Y. Saenz, et al., "Mechanisms of Antibiotic Resistance in Escherichia coli Isolates Recovered from Wild Animals," *Microbial Drug Resistance* 14 (2008): 71–77.

29. Costa et al. "Mechanisms of Antibiotic Resistance"; A. Smet, A. Martel, D. Persoons, et al., "Broad-Spectrum β-lactamases among Enterobacteriaceae of Animal Origin: Molecular Aspects, Mobility and Impact on Public Health," *FEMS Microbiology Reviews* 34 (2010): 295–316; S. Guenther, C. Ewers, and L. H. Wieler, "Extended-Spectrum Beta-lactamases Producing E. coli in Wildlife, yet Another Form of Environmental Pollution?" *Frontiers in Microbiology* 2 (2011): 1–13.

30. Guenther, Ewers, and Wieler, "Extended-Spectrum Beta-lactamases"; M. H. Nicolas-Chanoine, V. Leflon-Guibout, R. Demarty, et al., "Intercontinental Emergence of Escherichia coli Clone O25:H4-ST131 Producing CTX-M-15," *Journal of Antimicrobial Chemotherapy* 61 (2008): 273–81; C. Ewers, M. Grobbel, I. Stamm, et al., "Emergence of Human Pandemic O25:H4-ST131 CTX-M-15 Extended-spectrum Beta-lactamase-Producing Escherichia coli among Companion Animals," *Journal of Antimicrobial Chemotherapy* 65 (2010): 651–60.

31. J. Hernandez, J. Bonnedahl, I. Eliasson, et al., "Globally Disseminated Human Pathogenic Escherichia coli O25b-ST131 Clone, Harbouring blaCTX-M-15, Found in Glaucous-Winged Gull at Remote Commander Islands, Russia," *Environmental Microbiology Reports* 2 (2010): 329–32; Guenther, Ewers, and Wieler, "Extended-Spectrum Beta-lactamases."

32. Guenther, Ewers, and Wieler, "Extended-Spectrum Beta-lactamases"; M. J. Blaser, *Missing Microbes: How the Overuse of Antibiotics Is Fueling Our Modern Plagues* (New York: Henry Holt, 2014), pp. 5–6.

33. P. J. Turnbaugh, R. E. Ley, M. Hamady, et al., "The Human Microbiome Project: Exploring the Microbial Part of Ourselves in a Changing World," *Nature* 449 (2007): 804–10, www.ncbi.nlm.nih.gov/pmc/articles/PMC3709439/; Blaser, *Missing Microbes*, pp. 152–98.

34. A. K. Ortqvist, C. Lundholm, H. Kieler, et al., "Antibiotics in Fetal and Early Life and Subsequent Childhood Asthma: Nationwide Population Based Study with Sibling Analysis," *British Medical Journal* 349 (2014): g6979, doi: 10.1136/bmj.g6979.

35. J. L. Danzeisen, H. B. Kim, R. E. Isaacson, et al., "Modulations of the Chicken Cecal Microbiome and Metagenome in Response to Anticoccidial and Growth Promoter Treatment," *PLOS One* 6 (2011): e27949, www.plosone.org/article/info%3Adoi%2F10.1371%2Fjournal .pone.0027949#pone-0027949-g009. Recall that tylosin and virginiamycin are used as growth-promoting agents in poultry. Both have analogs in human medicine: tylosin/erythromycin and virginiamycin/quinupristin-dalfopristin.

36. T. Looft, H. K. Allen, B. L. Cantarel, et al., "Bacteria, Phages and Pigs: The Effects of In-feed Antibiotics on the Microbiome at Different Gut Locations," *ISME Journal* 8 (2014): 1566–76, www.nature.com/ismej/journal/v8/n8/full/ismej201412a.html. The doses were chlortetracycline 100 g per ton, sulfamethazine 100 g per ton, and penicillin 50 g per ton.

37. T. Looft, T. A. Johnson, H. K. Allen, et al., "In-feed Antibiotic Effects on the Swine Intestinal Microbiome," *Proceedings of the National Academy of Sciences* 109 (2012): 1691–1696, www.pnas.org/content/109/5/1691.full. According to the study authors, 50 years of using antibiotics in feed likely led to the high background level of resistance genes.

38. C. Liu, S. M. Finegold, Y. Song, et al., "Reclassification of *Clostridium coccoides, Ruminococcus hansenii, Ruminococcus hydrogenotrophicus, Ruminococcus luti, Ruminococcus productus* and *Ruminococcus schinkii* as *Blautia coccoides* gen. nov., comb. nov., *Blautia hansenii* comb. nov., *Blautia hydrogenotrophica* comb. nov., *Blautia luti* comb. mov., *Blautia producta* comb. nov., *Blautia schinkii* comb. nov. and description of *Blautia wexlerae* sp. Nov., isolated from human faeces," *International Journal of Systematic and Evolutionary Microbiology* 58 (2008): 1896–1902, http://ijs.sgmjournals.org/content/58/8/1896.full. Ruminococcus are Gram-positive, anaerobic gut microbes in animals and humans. Considerations are under way to reclassify it from Clostridia to a novel Blautia genus.

39. Looft et al. "In-feed Antibiotic Effects."

40. "Penicillin's Finder Assays Its Future," *New York Times,* June 26, 1945, p. 21. In 1945, at a dinner honoring Sir Alexander Fleming at New York City's Waldorf-Astoria, he cautioned the audience about the dangers of overusing antibiotics and predicted the development of resistant microbes.

41. V. M. D'Costa, E. Griffiths, and G. D. Wright, "Expanding the Soil Antibiotic Resistome: Exploring Environmental Diversity," *Current Opinion in Microbiology* 10, no. 5 (2007): 481–89; M. S. Butler, M. A. Blaskovich, and M. A. Cooper, "Antibiotics in the Clinical Pipeline in 2013," *Journal of Antibiotics* 66 (2013): 571–91; Infectious Disease Society of America (IDSA), "Combating Antimicrobial Resistance: Policy Recommendations to Save Lives," *Clinical Infectious Diseases* 52, Suppl. 5 (2011): S397–S428; B. Spellberg, J. H. Powers, E. P. Brass, et al., "Trends in Antimicrobial Drug Development: Implications for the Future," *Clinical Infectious Diseases* 38 (2004): 1279–86.

42. D. M. Shlaes, "The Abandonment of Antibacterials: Why and Wherefore?" *Current Opinion in Pharmacology* 3 (2003): 470–73; D. Hurley, "Why Are There So Few Blockbuster Drugs Invented Today?" *New York Times Magazine,* Innovations Issue, November 13, 2014, www.nytimes.com/2014/11/16/magazine/why-are-there-so-few-new-drugs-invented-today .html?smprod=nytcore-ipad&smid=nytcore-ipad-share&_r=0; Spellberg et al. "Trends in Antimicrobial Drug Development"; H. W. Boucher, G. H. Talbot, D. K. Benjamin Jr., et al., "10×'20 Progress—Development of New Drugs Active against Gram-Negative Bacilli: An Update from the Infectious Diseases Society of America," *Clinical Infectious Diseases* 56 (2013): 1685–94.

43. B. Alberts, M. W. Kirschner, S. Tilghman, et al., "Rescuing U.S. Biomedical Research from Its Systemic Flaws," *Proceedings of the National Academy of Sciences* 111 (2014): 5773–77, www.ncbi.nlm.nih.gov/pmc/articles/PMC4000813/pdf/pnas.201404402.pdf; J. A. Johnson, "Brief History of NIH Funding: Fact Sheet," *Congressional Research Service Report R43341*, December 23, 2013, http://fas.org/sgp/crs/misc/R43341.pdf.

44. Alberts et al., "Rescuing U.S. Biomedical Research." See also E. D. Brown, "Is the GAIN Act a Turning Point in New Antibiotic Discovery?" *Canadian Journal of Microbiology* 59 (2013): 153–56.

45. National Institutes of Health, Biomedical Research Workforce Working Group Report, June 14, 2012, http://acd.od.nih.gov/biomedical_research_wgreport.pdf; Alberts et al., "Rescuing U.S. Biomedical Research."

46. National Institutes of Health, "Fact Sheet: Impact of Sequestration on the National Institutes of Health," June 3, 2013, www.nih.gov/news/health/jun2013/nih-03.htm; N. Wade, "Rare Hits and Heaps of Misses to Pay For," *New York Times*, November 8, 2010, www.nytimes.com/2010/11/09/science/09wade.html?_r=0.

47. C. Nathan, "Antibiotic Resistance—Problems, Progress, and Prospects," *New England Journal of Medicine* 371 (2014): 1761–63; Boucher et al. "10×'20 Progress"; Butler, Blaskovich, and Cooper, "Antibiotics in the Clinical Pipeline"; Wade, "Rare Hits and Heaps of Misses."

48. T. Kirby, "Europe to Boost Development of New Antimicrobial Drugs," *Lancet* 379 (2012): 2229–30; See also Innovative Medicines Initiative, "Introducing IMI Mission," www.imi.europa.eu/content/mission.

49. Boucher et al., "10×'20 Progress"; B. E. Murray, "21st Century Cures: Examining Ways to Combat Antibiotic Resistance and Foster New Drug Development," written statement to the Energy and Commerce Committee, Health Subcommittee, U.S. House of Representatives, September 19, 2014, http://docs.house.gov/meetings/IF/IF14/20140919/102692/HHRG-113-IF14-Wstate-MurrayB-20140919.pdf; J. P. Gingrey, US Representative for Georgia's 11th congressional district since 2003, is a member of the Republican Party. R. E. Green, US Representative for Texas's 29th congressional district since 1993, is a member of the Democratic Party. Govtrack.us, S. 3187 (112th) Food and Drug Safety and Innovation Act of 2012. The bill became P.L. 112-144 on July 9, 2012. The GAIN Act designated new antibiotics as "Qualified Infectious Disease Products" (QIDPs), which are eligible for fast-track and priority review with the FDA. Once approved, QIDPs are free from generic competition for five years. J. Woodcock, "Three Encouraging Steps towards New Antibiotics," *FDAVoice*, September 23, 2014, http://blogs.fda.gov/fdavoice/index.php/tag/qualified-infectious-disease-product-qidp/.

50. Brown, "GAIN Act a Turning Point?"; Murray, "21st Century Cures"; Boucher et al., "10×'20 Progress."

51. President's Council of Advisors on Science and Technology (PCAST), "Report to the President on Combating Antibiotic Resistance," Executive Office of the President, September 2014, pp. 3, 28, 30, www.whitehouse.gov/sites/default/files/microsites/ostp/PCAST/pcast_carb_report_sept2014.pdf.

52. Ibid., p. 36; President George W. Bush signed the Pandemic and All-Hazards Preparedness Act of 2006, and it became Public Law No. 109-417. The law established the Biomedical Advanced Research and Development Authority to advance the development of medical countermeasures against biological, chemical, radiological, nuclear, and emerging infectious disease threats.

53. PCAST, "Report on Combating Antibiotic Resistance," pp. 37, 38–41.

54. Barry Eisenstein, MD, senior vice president, Scientific Affairs, Cubist Pharmaceuticals, e-mail communication, October 28, 2014. Cubist Pharmaceuticals was established in 1992 with its primary focus on developing novel antibiotics, On January 22, 2015, Cubist became a wholly owned subsidiary of Merck & Co. www.cubist.com/research-and-development/pipeline.

55. L. Dethlefsen, M. Mcfall-Ngai, and D. A. Relman, "An Ecological and Evolutionary Perspective on Human-Microbe Mutualism and Disease," *Nature* 449 (2007): 811–18; M. A. Riley, S. M. Robinson, C. M. Roy, et al., "Rethinking the Composition of a Rational Antibiotic Arsenal for the 21st Century," *Future Medicinal Chemistry* 5, no. 11 (2013): 1231–42, www.future-science.com/doi/abs/10.4155/fmc.13.79.

56. Riley et al "Rethinking Rational Antibiotic Arsenal."

57. F. W. Twort, "An Investigation on the Nature of Ultra-microscopic Viruses," *Lancet* (1915): 1241–43; F. D'Herelle, "An Invisible Antagonist Microbe of Dysentery Bacillus," *Comptes Rendus Hebdomadaires des Seances de L'academie des Sciences* (1917): 373–75; T. K. Lu and M. S. Koeris, "The Next Generation of Bacteriophage Therapy," *Current Opinion in Microbiology* 14 (2011): 524–31.

58. Lu and Koeris, "Next Generation of Bacteriophage Therapy"; J. J. Gill, T. Hollyer, and P. M. Sabour, "Bacteriophages and Phage-Derived Products as Antibacterial Therapeutics," *Expert Opinion on Therapeutic Patents* 17 (2007): 1341–50, http://informahealthcare.com/doi/abs/10.1517%2F13543776.17.11.1341.

59. In contrast, physicians currently use a "shotgun" approach with antibiotics. To save time, the infecting microbe is typically not identified. The clinician makes a "best guess" as to the likely causative disease agent. Not infrequently, this guess is incorrect, and the infecting microbe turns out to be a virus, for which antibiotics are inappropriate and useless.

60. Lu and Koeris, "Next Generation of Bacteriophage Therapy"; A. Sulakvelidze, Z. Alavidze, and J. G. Morris Jr., "Bacteriophage Therapy," *Antimicrobial Agents and Chemotherapy* 45 (2001): 649–59.

61. National Institutes of Health, "NIH Research Project Grant Program (R01)." R01 grants support health-related research. http://grants.nih.gov/grants/funding/r01.htm; NIH, Research Portfolio Online Reporting Tools (RePORT), http://report.nih.gov/; J. J. Gill, PhD, assistant professor, Department of Animal Science, Center for Phage Technology, Texas A&M University, e-mail communication, March 11, 2015. The three projects were 5R01AI057472-10, Isolation of New Phage Enzymes to Kill *B. anthracis;* 1R01GM110202-01A1, Structure, Function, and Engineering of Myovirus Phage CBA120 Tailspike Proteins; and 5R01AI081726-05, Structural Studies of Bacteriophage T4 and Their Potential Medical Applications.

62. Gill, e-mail communication, March 11, 2015.

63. Riley et al., "Rethinking Rational Antibiotic Arsenal."

64. Ibid. See also V. C. Kalia, "Quorum Sensing Inhibitors: An Overview," *Biotechnology Advances* 31 (2013): 224–45.

65. Kalia, "Quorum Sensing Inhibitors"; C. T. O'Loughlin, L. C. Miller, A. Siryaporn, et al., "A Quorum-Sensing Inhibitor Blocks Pseudomonas areuginosa Virulence and Biofilm Formation," *Proceedings of the National Academy of Sciences* 110 (2013): 17981–986, www.pnas.org/content/110/44/17981.full.

66. Kalia, "Quorum Sensing Inhibitors"; T. Defoirdt, N. Boon, P. Bossier, et al., "Disruption of Bacterial Quorum Sensing: An Unexplored Strategy to Fight Infections in Aquaculture," *Aquaculture* 240 (2004): 69–88; Defoirdt, Sorgeloos, and Bossier, "Alternatives to Antibiotics."

67. T. C. Lee, C. Frenette, D. Jayaraman, et al., "Antibiotic Self-stewardship: Trainee-Led Structured Antibiotic Time-Outs to Improve Antimicrobial Use," *Annals of Internal Medicine* 161 (2014): S53–S58, http://annals.org/article.aspx?articleID=1935743.

CHAPTER TEN: Conclusion

1. Food and Agriculture Organization (FAO), Animal Production and Health, "Sources of Meat," November 25, 2014, www.fao.org/ag/againfo/themes/en/meat/backgr_sources .html. Beef accounts for 22 percent of total intake.

2. V. Smil, *Feeding the World: A Challenge for the Twenty-First Century* (Cambridge, MA: MIT Press, 2002), pp. 156–57, 161–63. Dairy cattle, carp, and salmon are the most efficient species at converting feed to food.

3. B. Phalan, M. Onial, A. Balmford, et al., "Reconciling Food Production and Biodiversity Conservation: Land Sharing and Land Sparing Compared," *Science* 333 (2011): 1289–91.

4. A. E. van den Bogaard, N. Bruinsma, and E. E. Stobberingh, "The Effect of Banning Avoparcin on VRE Carrieage in the Netherlands," *Journal of Antimicrobial Chemotherapy* 46 (2000): 146–48; I. Klare, D. Badstubner, C. Konstabel, et al., "Decreased Incidence of VanA-type Vancomycin-Resistant Enterococci Isolated from Poultry Meat and from Fecal Samples of Humans in the Community after Discontinuation of Avoparcin Usage in Animal Husbandry," *Microbial Drug Resistance* 5 (1999): 45–52.

5. ECDC, EFSA, and EMA, "First Joint Report on the Integrated Analysis of the Consumption of Antimicrobial Agents and Occurrence of Antimicrobial Resistance in Bacteria from Humans and Food-Producing Animals," *EFSA Journal* 13 (2015): 1–114, doi: 10.2903 /j.efsa.2015.4006, www.efsa.europa.eu/fr/efsajournal/pub/4006.htm.

6. Ibid., p. 29, table 4; p. 32, fig. 4 a–c. The data was not completely harmonized. Some countries reported combined hospital and community antibiotic consumption. Others did not include antibiotic consumption in hospitals. In three countries, consumption was similar; in eight countries, animals consumed more than humans.

7. European Medicines Agency, "Trends in the Sales of Veterinary Antimicrobial Agents in Nine European Countries: Reporting Period: 2005–2009," September 15, 2011, www.ema .europa.eu/docs/en_GB/document_library/Report/2011/09/WC500112309.pdf. From 2005 to 2009, the EU collected veterinary antibiotic sales data from nine countries, four of which were considered large livestock producers. Denmark experienced an increase in therapeutic antibiotic use, particularly tetracycline use in pigs. The increase in tetracycline use led to an increase in tetracycline resistance in *Salmonella typhimurium* from pigs. The Czech Republic also experienced an increase in tetracycline use, but France and the Netherlands, the other two large livestock producers, experienced decreased tetracycline use.

8. European Medicines Agency, "Sales of Veterinary Antimicrobial Agents," pp. 37, 61–62, 59.

9. International Labor Organization, LABORSTA, UK 1991 price, Consumer Price Indices, main statistics annual, laborsta.ilo.org/STP/guest.

10. J. L. Dorne, M. L. Fernandez-Cruz, U. Bertelsen, et al., "Risk Assessment of Coccidiostatics during Feed Cross-Contamination: Animal and Human Health Aspects," *Toxicology and Applied Pharmacology* 270 (2013): 196–208, www.sciencedirect.com/science/article/pii /S0041008X10004795.

11. Executive Office of the President, PCAST, "Report to the President on Combating Antibiotic Resistance," September 2014, www.whitehouse.gov/sites/default/files/microsites /ostp/PCAST/pcast_carb_report_sept2014.pdf; White House, "National Strategy for Combating Antibiotic Resistant Bacteria," September 2014, www.whitehouse.gov/sites/default

/files/docs/carb_national_strategy.pdf; White House Office of the Press Secretary, "Fact Sheet: President's 2016 Budget Proposes Historic Investment to Combat Antibiotic-Resistant Bacteria to Protect Public Health," January 27, 2015, www.whitehouse.gov/the-press-office /2015/01/27/fact-sheet-president-s-2016-budget-proposes-historic-investment-combat-a.

12. American Presidency Project, Barack Obama, XLIV President of the United States, "677—Executive Order 13676—Combating Antibiotic-Resistant Bacteria," September 18, 2014, www.presidency.ucsb.edu/ws/index.php?pid=107546; White House Office of the Press Secretary, "President's 2016 Budget."

13. FDA, "FDA Secures Full Industry Engagement on Antimicrobial Resistance Strategy," June 30, 2014, www.fda.gov/AnimalVeterinary/NewsEvents/CVMUpdates/ucm403285.htm.

14. T. P. Van Boeckel, C. Brower, M. Gilbert, et al., "Global Trends in Antimicrobial Use in Food Animals," *Proceedings of the National Academy of Sciences* 2015: 1503141112v1– 201503141, www.pnas.org/content/early/2015/03/18/1503141112.abstract.

15. D. Kesmodel, "Meat Companies Go Antibiotics-Free as More Consumers Demand It," *Wall Street Journal,* November 3, 2014, www.wsj.com/articles/meat-companies-go-anti biotics-free-as-more-consumers-demand-it-1415071802; S. Strom, "McDonald's Moving to Limit Antibiotic Use in Chickens," *New York Times,* March 4, 2015, www.nytimes.com/2015 /03/05/business/mcdonalds-moving-to-antibiotic-free-chicken.html?emc=eta1&_r=0.

16. Kesmodel, "Meat Companies Go Antibiotics-Free"; M. Lipka, "Is Organic Chicken Worth the Price?" *Reuters,* July 17, 2014, www.reuters.com/article/2014/07/17/us-money -chicken-organic-idUSKBN0FM24Q20140717.

17. R. J. LeBlanc, P. Matthews, and R. P. Richard, "Global Atlas of Excreta, Wastewater Sludge, and Biosolids Management: Moving Forward the Sustainable and Welcome Uses of a Global Resource," United Nations Human Settlements Programme (UN-Habitat), 2008, Nairobi, Kenya, p. 3, http://esa.un.org/iys/docs/san_lib_docs/habitat2008.pdf; UNICEF, "Water and Sanitation," http://data.unicef.org/water-sanitation/sanitation.

18. A. Purss-Ustun, R. Bos, F. Gore, et al., "Safer Water, Better Health: Costs, Benefits and Sustainability of Interventions to Protect and Promote Health," World Health Organization, Geneva, Switzerland, 2008, pp. 7, 9, http://whqlibdoc.who.int/publications/2008/9789 241596435_eng.pdf?ua=1; R. S. Sharma, S. M. Kaul, and J. Sokhay, "Seasonal Fluctuations of Dengue Fever Vector, Aedes Aegypti (Diptera: Culicidae) in Delhi, India," *Southeast Asian Journal of Tropical Medicine and Public Health* 36 (2005): 186–90.

19. T. R. Burch, M. J. Sadowsky, and T. M. LaPara, "Fate of Antibiotic Resistance Genes and Class 1 Integrons in Soil Microcosms Following the Application of Treated Residual Municipal Wastewater Solids," *Environmental Science and Technology* 48 (2014): 5620–27, www.ncbi.nlm.nih.gov/pubmed/24762092; G. C. A. Amos, E. Gozzard, C. E. Carter, et al., "Validated Predictive Modeling of the Environmental Resistome," *International Society for Microbial Ecology Journal,* February 13, 2015, doi: 10.1038/ismej.2014.237, www.nature.com /ismej/journal/vaop/ncurrent/pdf/ismej2014237a.pdf.

20. National Human Genome Research Institute, "DNA Sequencing Costs: Data from the NHGRI Genome Sequencing Program (GSP)," Table Cost per Genome, www.genome.gov /sequencingcosts/. In July 2009, the cost was $108,065. In July 2014, the cost was $4,905; Executive Office of the President, "Report on Combating Antibiotic Resistance," pp. 4–5.

21. S. Coren, "Is That a Dog in Your Bed?" *Psychology Today,* September 23, 2014, www .psychologytoday.com/blog/canine-corner/201409/is-dog-in-your-bed.

22. E. Scott, S. Duty, and K. McCue, "A Critical Evaluation of Methicillin-Resistant Staphylococcus Aureus and Other Bacteria of Medical Interest on Commonly Touched Household Surfaces in Relation to Household Demographics," *American Journal of Infection Control* 37 (2009): 447–53, www.ncbi.nlm.nih.gov/pubmed/19361887.

23. S. Grant and C. W. Olsen, "Preventing Zoonotic Diseases in Immunocompromised Persons: The Role of Physicians and Veterinarians," *Emerging Infectious Diseases* 5 (1999): 159–63, wwwnc.cdc.gov/eid/article/5/1/99-0121_article.

24. F. Jabr, "It's Buggy Out There," *New York Times Magazine,* February 13, 2015, pp. 16–17, www.nytimes.com/2015/02/15/magazine/its-buggy-out-there.html?ref=magazine&_r=0; Human Microbiome Project Consortium, "Structure, Function and Diversity of the Healthy Human Microbiome," *Nature* 486 (2012): 207–14, www.nature.com/nature/journal/v486 /n7402/pdf/nature11234.pdf.

25. T. B. Stanton, "A Call for Antibiotic Alternatives Research," *Trends in Microbiology* 21 (2013): 111–13, www.sciencedirect.com/science/article/pii/S0966842X12001990.

26. I. Cho and M. J. Blaser, "The Human Microbiome: At the Interface of Health and Disease," *Nature Reviews/Genetics* 13 (2012): 260–70, www.nature.com/nrg/journal/v13/n4/abs /nrg3182.html. *Proteobacteria* are Gram negative, often purple colored, and include pathogens such as *Salmonella, E. coli,* and *Serratia marcescens. Actinobacteria* are Gram positive with a high guanine and cytosine content in their DNA; they are abundant in soil and seas and include *Streptomyces. Bacteroidetes* are Gram negative, anaerobic, and non-spore-forming and are abundant in sediments, soils, and oceans; they are common in the skin and intestines of mammals and include *Bacteroides. Firmicutes* are primarily Gram positive with low guanine and cytosine content in their DNA; they include *Clostridium* and *Bacillus.*

27. P. A. Thacker, "Alternatives to Antibiotics as Growth Promoters for Use in Swine Production: A Review," *Journal of Animal Science and Biotechnology* 4 (2013): 35, www.jasbsci .com/content/4/1/35.

28. M. Austin, M. Mellow, and W. M. Tierney, "Fecal Microbiota Transplantation in the Treatment of Clostridium difficile Infections," *American Journal of Medicine* 127 (2014): 479–83, www.ncbi.nlm.nih.gov/pubmed/24582877; L. J. Brandt, "Fecal Transplantation for the Treatment of Clostridium difficile Infection," *Gastroenterology and Hepatology* 8 (2012): 191–94, www.ncbi.nlm.nih.gov/pmc/articles/PMC3365524/.

29. K. A. Bauer, K. K. Perez, G. N. Forrest, et al., "Review of Rapid Diagnostic Tests Used by Antimicrobial Stewardship Programs," *Clinical Infectious Diseases* 59, Suppl. 3 (2014): S134–S145, http://cid.oxfordjournals.org/content/59/suppl_3/S134.short. These tests include polymerase chain reaction (PCR), multiplex PCR, nanoparticle probe technologies, and matrix-assisted laser desorption/ionization time-of-flight mass spectrometry (MALDI-TOF MS). G. N. Forrest, M.-C. Roghmann, L. S. Toombs, et al., "Peptide Nucleic Acid Fluorescent in Situ Hybridization for Hospital-Acquired Enterococcal Bacteremia: Delivering Earlier Effective Antimicrobial Therapy," *Antimicrobial Agents and Chemotherapy* 52 (2008): 3558–63. Peptide nucleic acid fluorescent in situ hybridization probes (PNA FISH) are DNA mimics that allow the identification of species-specific ribosomal RNA targets in bacteria. An FDA-approved test is commercially available for the rapid identification of *Enterococcus* species. One drop of blood from a positive blood culture containing Gram-positive cocci yields results in less than three hours, turning green for *Enterococcus faecalis,* red for other *Enterococcus* species, and no color if not an *Enterococcus* species.

30. R. P. N. Mishra, E. Oviedo-Orta, P. Prachi, et al., "Vaccines and Antibiotic Resistance," *Current Opinion in Microbiology* 15 (2012): 596–602, www.sciencedirect.com/science/article /pii/S1369527412001154; A. V. Gottberg, L. deGouveia, S. Tempia, et al., "Effects of Vaccination on Invasive Pneumococcal Disease in South Africa," *New England Journal of Medicine* 371 (2014): 1889–99, www.nejm.org/doi/pdf/10.1056/NEJMoa1401914; T. R. Talbot, K. A. Poehling, T. V. Hartert, et al., "Reductions in High Rates of Antibiotic-Nonsusceptible Invasive Pneumococcal Disease in Tennessee after Introduction of the Pneumococcal Conjugate Vaccine," *Clinical Infectious Disease* 39 (2004): 641–48, http://cid.oxfordjournals.org/content/39

/5/641.abstract?ijkey=c7d3e2ece236f6fd2b3c8ee44d14b624755e5703&keytype2=tf
_ipsecsha; K. P. Klugman, "Vaccination: A Novel Approach to Reduce Antibiotic Resistance,"
Clinical Infectious Diseases 39 (2004): 649–51, http://cid.oxfordjournals.org/content/39/5/649
.full.

31. J. D. Cherry, "Epidemic Pertussis in 2012—The Resurgence of a Vaccine-Preventable
Disease," *New England Journal of Medicine* 367 (2012): 785–87, www.nejm.org/doi/full/10.1056
/NEJMp1209051; D. E. Sugerman, A. E. Barskey, M. G. Delea, et al., "Measles Outbreak in a
Highly Vaccinated Population, San Diego, 2008: Role of the Intentionally Undervaccinated,"
Pediatrics 125 (2010): 747–55, http://pediatrics.aappublications.org/content/125/4/747.short; P
. A. Offit, "Why Are Pharmaceutical Companies Gradually Abandoning Vaccines?" *Health Affairs* 24 (2005): 622–30, http://content.healthaffairs.org/content/24/3/622.full.

32. A. N. Corallo, R. Croxford, D. C. Goodman, et al., "A Systematic Review of Medical
Practice Variation in OECD Countries," *Health Policy* 114 (2014): 5–14, www.healthpolicyjrnl
.com/article/S0168-8510(13)00215-7/abstract.

33. G. Mitsi, E. Jelastopulu, H. Basiaris, et al., "Patterns of Antibiotic Use among Adults
and Parents in the Community: A Questionnaire-Based Survey in a Greek Urban Population,"
International Journal of Antimicrobial Agents 25 (2005): 439–43, www.sciencedirect
.com/science/article/pii/S0924857905000580. One could argue that patient illness behavior
is as important, if not more important, than physician prescribing practices. Mitsi and colleagues developed a questionnaire-based survey and conducted 323 face-to-face interviews
with more than 170 adults in Greece, a country with very high antibiotic use rates. They
found that almost 75 percent of the adults surveyed admitted to using nonprescribed antibiotics and almost half discontinued therapy early. Approximately 55 percent admitted to
using leftover antibiotics and more than 10 percent did not follow dosage instructions. See
also E. Sabuncu, J. David, C. Bernede-Bauduin, et al., "Significant Reduction of Antibiotic
Use in the Community after a Nationwide Campaign in France, 2002–2007," *PLOS Medicine*
6, no. 6 (2009): e1000084, http://journals.plos.org/plosmedicine/article?id=10.1371/journal
.pmed.1000084. In 2001 France implemented a "Keep Antibiotics Working" initiative in an
effort to reduce unnecessary antibiotic use. The main component was a public education
campaign, "Antibiotics Are not Automatic," that was launched one year later. A before-and-
after evaluation of the program, using data from the French National Health Insurance
database and national disease surveillance system, found that use of all major classes of
antibiotics, except quinolones, decreased in all 22 French regions. The greatest decrease in
prescription rates, by about 33 percent compared to precampaign levels, was in children
ages 6 to 15.

34. ECDC, "European Surveillance of Antibiotic Consumption (ESAC-Net)," www.ecdc
.europa.eu/en/activities/surveillance/ESAC-Net/Pages/index.aspx; K. Sinha, "India Is the
World's Largest Consumer of Antibiotics," *Times of India,* July 14, 2014, http://timesofindia
.indiatimes.com/india/India-is-the-worlds-largest-consumer-of-antibiotics/articleshow
/38348426.cms.

35. IMS Health, company website, www.imshealth.com/portal/site/imshealth.

36. European Medicines Agency, "European Surveillance of Veterinary Antimicrobial Consumption (ESVAC)," www.ema.europa.eu/ema/index.jsp?curl=pages/regulation/document
_listing/document_listing_000302.jsp; European Medicines Agency, "Sales of Veterinary Antimicrobial Agents."

37. FDA, "ADUFA Reports: Antimicrobial Animal Drug Distribution Reports," www.fda
.gov/ForIndustry/UserFees/AnimalDrugUserFeeActADUFA/ucm042896.htm.

38. CDC, "Get Smart: Know When Antibiotics Work," www.cdc.gov/getsmart/index
.html; R. Colgan and J. H. Powers, "Appropriate Antimicrobial Prescribing: Approaches That

Limit Antibiotic Resistance," *American Family Physician* 64 (2001): 999–1004, www.aafp.org /afp/2001/0915/p999.html; N. Safdar, T. G. Tape, B. C. Fox, et al., "Factors Affecting Antibiotic Prescribing for Acute Respiratory Infection by Emergency Physicians," *Health* 6 (2014): 774–80, www.scirp.org/journal/PaperInformation.aspx?PaperID=44177#.VOoYEFtATB4.

39. CDC, "About the Get Smart Campaign," www.cdc.gov/getsmart/campaign-materials /about-campaign.html.

40. FDA, "Guidance for Industry #209: The Judicious Use of Medically Important Antimicrobial Drugs in Food-Producing Animals," April 13, 2012, www.fda.gov/downloads /AnimalVeterinary/GuidanceComplianceEnforcement/GuidanceforIndustry/UCM216936 .pdf; CDC, "Guide to Infection Prevention for Outpatient Setting: Minimum Expectations for Safe Care," www.cdc.gov/HAI/settings/outpatient/outpatient-care-guidelines.html; CDC, "Healthcare Infection Control Practices Advisory Committee (HICPAC)," General Guidelines, www.cdc.gov/hicpac/pubs.html; AVMA, "Judicious Therapeutic Use of Antimicrobials," www.avma.org/KB/Policies/Pages/Judicious-Therapeutic-Use-of-Antimicrobials.aspx. The CDC reportedly provided input for these recommendations. NASPHV, "NASPHV Compendia and Recommendations. Model Infection Control Plan for Veterinary Practices," www.nasphv.org/documentsCompendia.html.

41. R. Harris, "When Scientists Give Up," *All Things Considered,* National Public Radio, September 9, 2014, www.npr.org/blogs/health/2014/09/09/345289127/when-scientists-give -up?refresh=true.

42. B. Alberts, M. W. Kirschner, S. Tilghman, et al., "Rescuing U.S. Biomedical Research from Its Systemic Flaws," *Proceedings of the National Academy of Sciences* 111 (2014): 5773–77, www.pnas.org/content/111/16/5773.full.

43. National Institutes of Health, *Veterinary-Scientists as Participants in the NIH-Funded Workforce in Physician-Scientist Workforce (PSW) Report 2014,* chap. 5, http://report.nih.gov /workforce/psw/veterinary_scientists.aspx.

44. Executive Office of the President, PCAST, "Report on Combating Antibiotic Resistance," p. 35; E. J. Emanuel, "How to Develop New Antibiotics," *New York Times,* February 24, 2015, www.nytimes.com/2015/02/24/opinion/how-to-develop-new-antibiotics.html?ref=opinion.

45. W. Diller, "How Durata Plans to Market Its Expensive New Antibiotic," *Forbes,* June 5, 2014, www.forbes.com/sites/wendydiller/2014/06/05/how-durata-plans-to-market-its -expensive-new-antibiotic/; A. T. Clyde, L. Bockstedt, J. A. Farkas, et al., "Experience with Medicare's New Technology Add-on Payment Program," *Health Affairs* 27 (2008): 1632–41, http:// content.healthaffairs.org/content/27/6/1632.full. Congress passed the Medicare, Medicaid, and State Children's Health Insurance Program (SCHIP) Benefits Improvement and Protection Act (BIPA), which included in H.R. 4577 the Consolidated Appropriations Act of 2001. President Bill Clinton signed it into law on December 21, 2000. www.govtrack.us/congress/bills /106/hr4577. The law mandated an additional payment under the inpatient payment system.

46. J. Scott, "Hospital Medicare Pay Down Slightly in 2015: CMS Makes Quality Program and Other Changes in Its FY 2015 Hospital Inpatient Proposed Rule," August 4, 2014, www.appliedpolicy.com/2014/08/fy15-hospital-ipps-final-rule/. CMS approved three of five new technology add-on payments (NTAP) and denied two for failing to meet substantial clinical improvement criteria.

47. Executive Office of the President, PCAST, "Report on Combating Antibiotic Resistance," p. 36.

48. D. Kriebel, J. Tickner, P. Epstein, et al., "The Precautionary Principle in Environmental Science," *Environmental Health Perspectives* 109 (2001): 871–76, www.ncbi.nlm.nih.gov /pmc/articles/PMC1240435/. See also National Institute for Animal Agriculture, "White Paper: The Precautionary Principle and Animal Agriculture," 2014 Annual Conference,

Omaha, Nebraska, April 1–2, 2014, p. 5, www.animalagriculture.org/Resources/Documents
/Conf%20-%20Symp/Conferences/2014%20Annual%20Conference/FINAL_May%2016
_Precautionary%20Principle%20White%20Paper.pdf; S. M. Gardiner, "A Core Precaution-
ary Principle," *Journal of Political Philosophy* 14 (2006): 33–60, www.public.iastate.edu
/~jwcwolf/Papers/Gardiner%20on%20Precautionary%20Principle.pdf.

49. C. Starr, "The Precautionary Principle versus Risk Analysis," *Risk Analysis* 23 (2003):
1–3, http://onlinelibrary.wiley.com/doi/10.1111/1539-6924.00285/full; National Institute
for Animal Agriculture, "Precautionary Principle and Animal Agriculture," p. 5.

50. M. Winerip, "The Death and Afterlife of Thalidomide," *New York Times,* September 23,
2013, www.nytimes.com/2013/09/23/booming/the-death-and-afterlife-of-thalidomide.html.
In the 1950s, a German company developed and marketed thalidomide as a treatment for
morning sickness in pregnant women. Thousands of children were born with severe birth
defects, including flipperlike arms and legs. Thanks to the concerns of Dr. Frances Kelsey,
an FDA medical officer, the United States avoided the tragedy by not approving the drug. I. M.
Vilas-Boas and C. P. Tharp, "The Drug Approval Process in the U.S., Europe, and Japan," *Journal of Managed Care Pharmacy* 3 (1997): 459–65, http://amcp.org/WorkArea/DownloadAsset
.aspx?id=5884.

After the thalidomide tragedy of the early 1960s, Congress passed the Kefauver-Harris
Amendments, which made the FDA drug approval process even more stringent. As a result,
the United States typically lagged behind Europe in approving drugs. J. A. Lisman and J. F. F.
Lekkerkerker, "Four Decades of European Medicines Regulation: What Have They Brought
Us?" *International Journal of Risk and Safety in Medicine* 17 (2005): 73–79, www.lismanll.nl
/files/documents/2005%20lisman%20lekkerkerker.pdf.

Immediately after the thalidomide tragedy, several European countries responded by
establishing their own regulatory bodies that required premarketing approval of medicines.
The European drug approval process during the time of thalidomide was virtually nonexistent, and several decades passed before the European Union implemented a drug evaluation
and approval process as stringent as that of the United States. "Council Directive 65/65/EEC
of 26 January 1965 on the Approximation of Provisions Laid Down by Law, Regulation or
Administrative Action Relating to Proprietary Medicinal Products," http://eur-lex.europa.eu
/LexUriServ/LexUriServ.do?uri=CELEX:31965L0065:EN:HTML. In January 1965 Europe
passed Council Directive 65/65; Lisman and Lekkerkerker, "Four Decades of Medicines Regulation." It was one of the first European legislative attempts to harmonize premarketing authorization of medicines. Its scope was limited to proprietary medicinal products; generic
drugs were not included, and blood products, radiopharmaceuticals, homeopathic medicines,
and vaccines had exemptions. European Medicines Agency, "20th Anniversary of EMA,"
www.ema.europa.eu/ema/index.jsp?curl=pages/about_us/general/general_content_000628
.jsp&mid=WC0b01ac058087addd.

In 1975 Europe passed a second directive, which extended the scope of European legislation on additional aspects of regulating medicines. The Committee on Proprietary Medicinal Products (CPMP) and the Pharmaceutical Committee were established, but their roles
were only advisory. They did not have decision-making authority. Europe also passed Directive 75/318/EEC, which included an annex that required data to be collected and submitted
before an application for drug approval could be made. From 1985 to 1995, CPMP's role became more prominent. In 1987 Council Directive 87/22/EEC was passed; it authorized the
first European procedure for the authorization of medicines. A single European market was
established in 1992 and came into force in 1995. An extensive review in 2001 led to more
harmonization, a stronger centralized approach, transparency, and pharmaceutical vigi-

lance. The European Medicines Agency (EMA), the EU equivalent to the FDA, was not established until 1995.

51. M. Bittman, "Stop Making Us Guinea Pigs," *New York Times,* March 25, 2015, www .nytimes.com/2015/03/25/opinion/stop-making-us-guinea-pigs.html?ref=opinion.

52. M. Woolhouse and J. Farrar, "An Intergovernmental Panel on Antimicrobial Resistance," *Nature* 509 (2014): 555–57.

53. World Health Organization, 68th World Health Assembly, Agenda Item 15.1, Global action plan on antimicrobial resistance, draft resolution with amendments resulting from informal consultations, May 25, 2015, Geneva, Switzerland, http://apps.who.int/gb/ebwha /pdf_files/WHA68/A68_ACONF1Rev1-en.pdf?ua=1.

54. United Nations, Framework Convention on Climate Change, "Background on the UNFCCC: The International Response to Climate Change," http://unfccc.int/essential _background/items/6031.php. The Kyoto Protocol was the product of two years of negotiations to strengthen the global response to climate change.

55. White House, "Fact Sheet: Obama Administration Releases National Action Plan to Combat Antibiotic-Resistant Bacteria," March 27, 2015, www.whitehouse.gov/the-press -office/2015/03/27/fact-sheet-obama-administration-releases-national-action-plan -combat-ant; White House, "National Action Plan for Combating Antibiotic-Resistant Bacteria," March 2015, www.whitehouse.gov/sites/default/files/docs/national_action_plan_for _combating_antibotic-resistant_bacteria.pdf; B. Estabrook, "Denmark's Drug-Free Pigs," *New York Times,* April 3, 2015, www.nytimes.com/2015/04/03/opinion/denmarks-drug-free -pigs.html?emc=eta1&_r=0.

56. J. Gillis and M. Richtel, "Beneath California Crops, Groundwater Crisis Grows," *New York Times,* April 5, 2015, www.nytimes.com/2015/04/06/science/beneath-california-crops -groundwater-crisis-grows.html?hp&action=click&pgtype=Homepage&module=first -column-region&region=top-news&WT.nav=top-news&_r=0. California's drought has become so severe that Governor Jerry Brown has imposed mandatory cuts in urban water use. I. Perez, "Climate Change and Rising Food Prices Heightened Arab Spring," *Scientific American,* March 4, 2013, www.scientificamerican.com/article/climate-change-and-rising -food-prices-heightened-arab-spring/.

57. M. Specter, "Test-Tube Burgers," *New Yorker,* May 23, 2011, www.newyorker.com /magazine/2011/05/23/test-tube-burgers; A. Halloran and P. Vantomme, "The Contribution of Insects to Food Security, Livelihoods and the Environment," FAO, 2013, www.fao.org /docrep/018/i3264e/i3264e00.pdf; FAO, "Insects for Food and Feed, www.fao.org/forestry /edibleinsects/en/.

Appendix A

1. Subcommittee chairs are listed for subcommittee hearings.

2. Penicillin Amendment of 1945, chap. 281, sec. 3, pp. 463–64.

3. U.S. General Accounting Office, Statement of Gregory C. Ahart, director, Human Resources Division, before the Subcommittee on Oversight and Investigations, House Committee on Interstate and Foreign Commerce on Food and Drug Administration's Regulation of Antibiotics Used in Animal Feeds, September 19, 1977, www.gao.gov/assets/100/98536.pdf.

4. H.R. 7285, 96th Cong., Antibiotics Preservation Act of 1980, www.govtrack.us /congress/bills/96/hr7285.

5. H.R. 6370, Antibiotic Protection Act of 1984, 98th Cong., Congress.gov.

6. S. D. Holmberg, M. T. Osterholm, K. A. Senger, and M. L. Cohen, "Drug-Resistant Salmonella from Animals Fed Antimicrobials," *New England Journal of Medicine* 311 (1984):

617–22; 98th Cong., 2nd Sess., Subcommittee on Investigations and Oversight, Committee on Science and Technology, U.S. House of Representatives, December 18, 1984, pp. 9–79.

7. H.R. 616, 99th Cong., Antibiotic Protection Act of 1985, www.govtrack.us/congress /bills/99/hr616.

8. GAO, Food Safety and Quality, "FDA Needs Stronger Controls over the Approval Process for New Animal Drugs," January 1992, GAO/RCED-92-63, www.gao.gov/assets/220 /215490.pdf.

9. FDA, Animal and Veterinary, Animal Medicinal Drug Use Clarification Act of 1994, www.fda.gov/AnimalVeterinary/GuidanceComplianceEnforcement/ActsRulesRegulations /ucm085377.htm.

10. H.R. 5056, 103rd Cong., Animal Medicinal Drug Use Clarification Act of 1994, www .govtrack.us/congress/bills/103/s340.

11. Office of Technology Assessment, *Impacts of Antibiotic Resistant Bacteria,* U.S. Congress, OTA-H-629 (Washington, DC: Government Printing Office, 1995), p. 159, table 7-2.

12. H.R. 2508, 104th Cong., Animal Drug Availability Act of 1996, www.govtrack.us /congress/bills/104/hr2508.

13. FDA, Animal and Veterinary, Animal Drug Availability Act of 1996, www.fda.gov /AnimalVeterinary/GuidanceComplianceEnforcement/ActsRulesRegulations/ucm105940 .htm.

14. CDC, Interagency Task Force on Antimicrobial Resistance, "About ITFAR" www.cdc .gov/drugresistance/itfar/about.html.

15. GAO, Food Safety, "The Agricultural Use of Antibiotics and Its Implications for Human Health," April 1999, GAO/RCED-99-74, www.gao.gov/assets/230/227223.pdf.

16. GAO, Antimicrobial Resistance, "Data to Assess Public Health Threat from Resistant Bacteria Are Limited," April 1999, GAO/HEHS/NSIAD/RCED-99-132, www.gao.gov/assets /230/227221.pdf.

17. H.R. 3266 Preservation of Essential Antibiotics for Human Diseases Act of 1999, www .congress.gov/bill/106th-congress/house-bill/3266.

18. NIH, Office of Legislative Policy and Analysis, 107th Congress, Antibiotic Resistance Prevention Act of 2001, http://olpa.od.nih.gov/legislation/107/pendinglegislation/antibi oticresistance.asp.

19. H.R. 1260, 108th Cong., Animal Drug User Fee Act of 2003, www.govtrack.us /congress/bills/108/hr1260.

20. GAO, "Federal Agencies Need to Better Focus Efforts to Address Risk to Humans from Antibiotic Use in Animals," GAO-04-490, April 2004, www.gao.gov/assets/250 /242186.pdf.

21. S. 15, 108th Cong., Project BioShield Act of 2004, www.govtrack.us/congress/bills /108/s15.

22. S. 3678, 109th Cong., Pandemic and All-Hazards Preparedness Act, www.govtrack.us /congress/bills/109/s3678.

23. H.R. 3580, 110th Cong., Food and Drug Administration Amendments Act of 2007, www.govtrack.us/congress/bills/110/hr3580/text.

24. Strategies to Address Antimicrobial Resistance Act, www.govtrack.us/congress/bills /110/s2313/text.

25. H.R. 6432, 110th Cong., Animal Drug User Fee Amendments of 2008, www.govtrack .us/congress/bills/110/hr6432.

26. GAO Report, "Food and Drug Administration's Regulation of Antibiotics Used in Animal Feeds," September 19, 1977, p. 8, www.gao.gov/assets/100/98536.pdf.

27. 111th Cong., 2nd Sess., *Antibiotic Resistance and the Threat to Public Health: Hearing before the Subcommittee on Health of the Committee on Energy and Commerce*, U.S. House of Representatives, April 28, 2010, Serial No. 111–15, p. 12.

28. *Promoting the Development of Antibiotics and Ensuring Judicious Use in Humans: Hearing before the Subcommittee on Health of the Committee on Energy and Commerce*, U.S. House of Representatives, 111th Cong., June 9, 2010, testimony by Barry I. Eisenstein, senior vice president, Cubist Pharmaceuticals, p. 131.

29. H.R. 6331, 111th Cong., Generating Antibiotic Incentives Now Act of 2010, www .govtrack.us/congress/bills/111/hr6331.

30. GAO, Antibiotic Resistance, "Data Gaps Will Remain Despite HHS Taking Steps to Improve Monitoring," June 2011, GAO-11-406, www.gao.gov/assets/320/319110.pdf.

31. H.R. 2182, 112th Cong., Generating Antibiotic Incentives Now Act of 2011, www .govtrack.us/congress/bills/112/hr2182.

32. S. 2373, 112th Cong., National Sustainable Offshore Aquaculture Act of 2011, www .govtrack.us/congress/bills/112/hr2373.

33. GAO, Antibiotic Resistance, "Agencies Have Made Limited Progress Addressing Antibiotic Use in Animals," September 2011, GAO-11-801, www.gao.gov/assets/330/323090.pdf.

34. S. 1529, 112th Cong., Foodborne Illness Reduction Act of 2011, www.govtrack.us /congress/bills/112/s1529.

35. GAO, Antibiotics, "FDA Needs to Do More to Ensure That Drug Labels Contain Up-to-Date Information," January 2012, GAO-12-218, www.gao.gov/assets/590/588022.pdf.

36. S. 3187, 112th Cong., Food and Drug Administration Safety and Innovation Act, www.govtrack.us/congress/bills/112/s3187.

37. H.R. 820, Delivering Antimicrobial Transparency in Animals Act of 2013, www .govtrack.us/congress/bills/113/hr820.

38. S. 1256, Preventing Antibiotic Resistance Act of 2013, www.govtrack.us/congress /bills/113/s1256.

39. S. 1502, Safe Meat and Poultry Act of 2013, www.govtrack.us/congress/bills/113/s1502.

Appendix B

1. 79th Cong., 1st Sess., Public Laws, chap. 281, July 6, 1945, pp. 463–64; *Federal Register* 3647–48 (April 28, 1951).

2. *Federal Register* 31, no. 163 (August 23, 1966).

3. FDA Guidance for Industry #152, "Evaluating the Safety of Antimicrobial New Animal Drugs with Regard to Their Microbiological Effects on Bacteria of Human Health Concern," October 2003, p. 6, www.fda.gov/downloads/AnimalVeterinary/GuidanceComplianceEnforcement/GuidanceforIndustry/UCM052519.pdf.

4. GAO Report, "Food and Drug Administration's Regulation of Antibiotics Used in Animal Feeds," September 19, 1977, www.gao.gov/assets/100/98536.pdf.

5. *Federal Register* 68, no. 153 (August 8, 2003): 47273.

6. GAO Report, "Food and Drug Administration's Regulation.

7. Ibid., p. 4.

8. Ibid., p. 5.

9. Ibid., p. 12.

10. Ibid., p. 9.

11. Ibid., p. 11.

12. FDA Guidance for Industry #152, "Evaluating the Safety of Antimicrobial New Animal Drugs with Regard to Their Microbiological Effects on Bacteria of Human Health

Concern," October 2003, pp. 6–7, www.fda.gov/downloads/AnimalVeterinary/Guidance ComplianceEnforcement/GuidanceforIndustry/UCM052519.pdf.

13. Ibid., pp. 7–8; U.S. Bureau of Veterinary Medicine, U.S. Public Health Service, Seattle–King County Department of Health, "Surveillance of the Flow of Salmonella and Campylobacter in a Community," Seattle–King County Department of Public Health, 1984, p. 3.

14. B. E. Murray, "21st Century Cures: Examining Ways to Combat Antibiotic Resistance and Foster New Drug Development," written statement to the Energy and Commerce Committee, Health Subcommittee, U.S. House of Representatives, September 19, 2014, http://docs.house .gov/meetings/IF/IF14/20140919/102692/HHRG-113-IF14-Wstate-MurrayB-20140919.pdf.

15. CDC, Interagency Task Force on Antimicrobial Resistance, Public Health Action Plan 2001, www.cdc.gov/drugresistance/pdf/public-health-action-plan-combat-antimicrobial -resistance.pdf.

16. FDA, Animal & Veterinary Antimicrobial Resistance website, www.fda.gov/Animal Veterinary/GuidanceComplianceEnforcement/GuidanceforIndustry/ucm123614.htm.

17. A. Franklin, J. Acar, F. Anthony, et al., "Antimicrobial Resistance: Harmonization of National Antimicrobial Resistance Monitoring and Surveillance Programmes in Animals and in Animal-Derived Food," *Scientific and Technical Review, Office International Epizooties* 20 (2001): 859–70, www.oie.int/doc/ged/D2010.PDF.

18. FDA Guidance for Industry #152, "Evaluating the Safety of Antimicrobial New Animal Drugs with Regard to Their Microbiological Effects on Bacteria of Human Health Concern," October 2003, www.fda.gov/downloads/AnimalVeterinary/GuidanceComplianceEnforcement /GuidanceforIndustry/UCM052519.pdf.

19. FDA Guidance for Industry #144, "Pre-approval Information for Registration of New Veterinary Medicinal Products for Food-Producing Animals with Respect to Antimicrobial Resistance," April 2004, www.fda.gov/downloads/AnimalVeterinary/GuidanceCompliance Enforcement/GuidanceforIndustry/UCM052524.pdf.

20. Food and Drug Administration, "FDA Announces Final Decision about Veterinary Medicine," July 28, 2005, pp. 5–48, www.fda.gov/NewsEvents/Newsroom/PressAnnouncements /2005/ucm108467.

21. Veterinary Feed Directive, "Advanced Notice of Proposed Rulemaking," *Federal Register,* March 29, 2010, www.federalregister.gov/articles/2010/03/29/2010-6872/veterinary-feed -directive.

22. FDA, Drugs, "Antibacterial Resistance and Diagnostic Device and Drug Development Research for Bacterial Diseases," Public Workshop, July 26–27, 2010, www.fda.gov/Drugs /NewsEvents/ucm211146.htm. Speaker: Dr. Lauri Hicks, medical director of Get Smart, CDC. Transcript, July 26, 2010, pp. 77–100, www.fda.gov/downloads/Drugs/NewsEvents /UCM226072.pdf.

23. Ibid., p. 156.

24. Ibid., p. 157.

25. FDA Guidance for Industry #209, "The Judicious Use of Medically Important Antimicrobial Drugs in Food-Producing Animals," April 2012, www.fda.gov/downloads/AnimalVeterinary/GuidanceComplianceEnforcement/GuidanceforIndustry/UCM216936.pdf.

26. Ibid.

27. FDA Guidance for Industry #213, "New Animal Drugs and New Animal Drug Combination Products Administered in or on Medicated Feed or Drinking Water of Food-Producing Animals: Recommendations for Drug Sponsors for Voluntarily Aligning Product Use Conditions with GFI #209," December 2013, www.fda.gov/downloads/AnimalVeterinary /GuidanceComplianceEnforcement/GuidanceforIndustry/UCM299624.pdf.

28. Ibid.

Appendix C

1. National Research Council (NRC), Committee on Animal Health, Agricultural Board, *A Nationwide System for Animal Health Surveillance* (Washington DC: National Academy of Sciences, 1974).

2. GAO Report, "Food and Drug Administration's Regulation of Antibiotics Used in Animal Feeds," September 19, 1977, p. 2, www.gao.gov/assets/100/98536.pdf.

3. NRC, Committee on Animal Health, Agricultural Board, *Nationwide System for Animal Health Surveillance*.

4. NRC, *The Effects on Human Health of Subtherapeutic Use of Antimicrobials in Animal Feeds* (Washington DC: The National Academies Press, 1980), p. 53.

5. Institute of Medicine (IOM), *Report of a Study: Human Health Risks with the Subtherapeutic Use of Penicillin or Tetracyclines in Animal Feed* (Washington, DC: National Academy Press, 1988), pp. 1–10, www.fda.gov/ohrms/dockets/dailys/03/Aug03/081403/03n-0324-bkg0001 -05-tab-4-01-vol2.pdf.

6. IOM, *Emerging Infections: Microbial Threats to Health in the United States* (Washington, DC: National Academy Press, 1992), pp. 11–12, www.nap.edu/openbook.php?record_id=2008.

7. IOM, *Antimicrobial Resistance: Issues and Options,* Forum on Emerging Infections, Workshop Report (Washington, DC: National Academy Press, 1998), p. 4, www.nap.edu /openbook.php?record_id=6121&page=R2.

8. Ibid., p. 94.

9. NRC, *The Use of Drugs in Food Animals: Benefits and Risks* (Washington, DC: National Academies Press, 1999), pp. 7–10.

10. Institute of Medicine, *Microbial Threats to Health: Emergence, Detection, and Response* (Washington, DC: National Academies Press, 2003), p. 15.

11. IOM, *Antibiotic Resistance: Implications for Global Health and Novel Intervention Strategies,* Workshop Summary (Washington, DC: National Academies Press, 2010).

12. H. G. Wegener, "Antibiotic Resistance—Linking Human and Animal Health," in IOM, *Improving Food Safety through a One Health Approach,* Workshop Summary (Washington, DC: National Academies Press, 2015), appendix A15, pp. 331–49.

13. NRC, *Technological Challenges in Antibiotic Discovery and Development,* Workshop Summary (Washington, DC: National Academies Press, 2014).

Index

DATE DUE

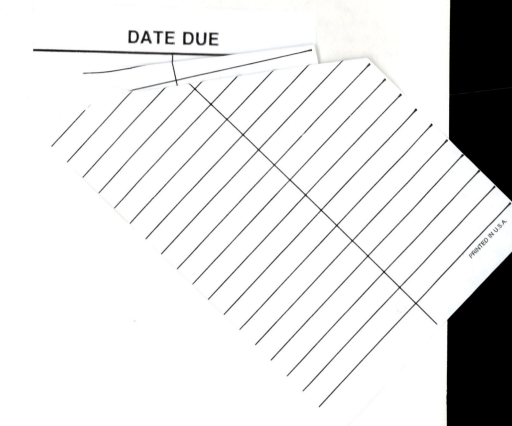

PRINTED IN U.S.A.